CRYSTAL BODY GRIDS

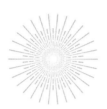

In *Crystal Body Grids* McAllister describes perfectly the basic principle of healing with crystals similar to the way I myself have worked with patients and taught healing for decades. The energy comes first and the body follows. Her book explains clearly the practical methods that can be used directly to treat many different problems, and it is a great work for anyone who is keen to take care of their own health, and that of others, in a wider sense.

Ewald Kliegel, author of *Crystal Wands: For Massage Therapy, Reflexology, and Energy Medicine* and the *Body Healing Cards*

Crystal Body Grids offers detailed instructions for using crystals for energetic healing. McAllister provides specific instructions for crystal alignments, chakra awareness, and physical healing, complementing traditional healing beautifully. The photos and diagrams give you everything you need to integrate these body, mind, and spirit practices into your life. What a beautiful and comprehensive book!

Margaret Ann Lembo, author of *The Essential Guide to Crystals, Minerals and Stones* and *Chakra Awakening: Transform Your Reality Using Crystals, Colors, Aromatherapy and the Power of Positive Thought*

Disclaimer

It is my fervent hope that you will very much enjoy all the practical crystal wisdom outlined in this book. If you have health concerns, I recommend always consulting your doctor prior to beginning to work with crystals. Crystals are noninvasive and therefore may be used positively alongside medical treatment. For your own reassurance, however, always check with your doctor first.

Please do not combine crystal use with recreational drugs and/or alcohol. Positive use of crystals seeks to balance the four lower bodies, and introducing toxins to the body/energy field is counterproductive.

Always take care using crystals around children and babies. Keep small crystals well out of their reach.

I hope this clarifies the safe and positive use of crystals.

Sharon L. McAllister

CRYSTAL BODY GRIDS

56 GEMSTONE LAYOUTS
FOR ENERGY HEALING

SHARON L. McALLISTER

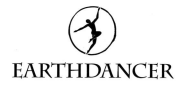

EARTHDANCER

AN INNER TRADITIONS IMPRINT

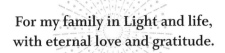

**For my family in Light and life,
with eternal love and gratitude.**

First edition 2024

Crystal Body Grids
56 Gemstone Layouts for Energy Healing
Sharon L. McAllister

This English edition © 2024 Earthdancer GmbH
Editing by JMS books LLP (www.jmseditorial.com)

Cover design: DesignIsIdentity.com
Cover illustration: Karola Sieber; model: Dilara Demir
Typesetting and layout: DesignIsIdentity.com
Typesetting body diagrams: Chris Bell, cbdesign
Typeset in Whitman and Myriad

Printed and bound in China by Reliance Printing Co., Ltd.

Cataloging-in-Publication Data for this title is available from the
Library of Congress

ISBN 979-8-88850-086-6 (print)
ISBN 979-8-88850-087-3 (ebook)

Published by Earthdancer, an imprint of Inner Traditions
www.earthdancerbooks.com, www.innertraditions.com

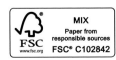

Contents

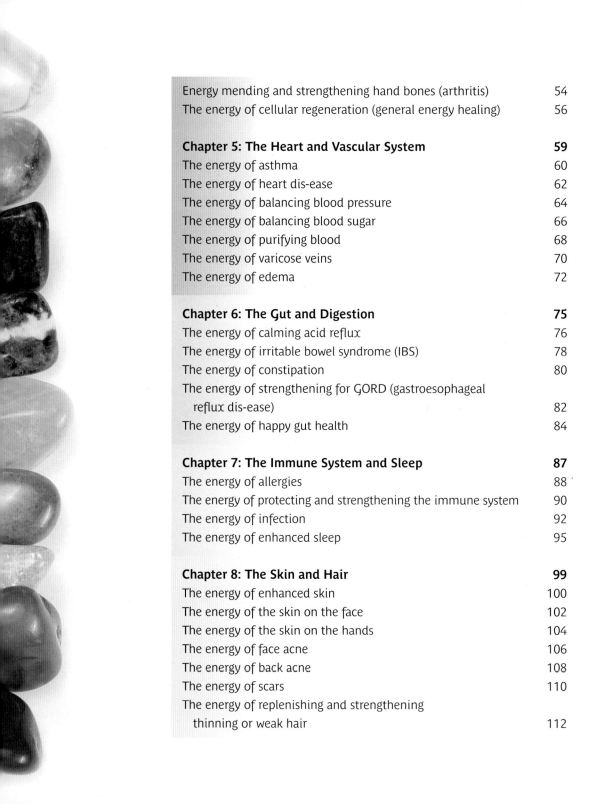

Introduction

My first book, *Awakening Your Crystals*, is a general introduction to getting started with crystals for everyday use—for yourself, your family and friends, and your environment. I place particular focus on eight powerful, readily available crystals that can be used to perform amazing, energetic multitasking on a wide variety of the challenges that we all regularly encounter.

Crystal Body Grids: 56 Gemstone Layouts for Energy Healing goes deeper, offering more practical, in-depth information on using crystals on a daily basis. It is a guide to how crystal energy can help with everyday *physical* well-being challenges and occurrences. We live in challenging times in which, as well as consulting medical professionals, we need to take greater responsibility for supporting our own health. Engaging with positive energy, particularly in the form of crystals, is a way to empower our well-being in all areas of our lives. *Crystal Body Grids: 56 Gemstone Layouts for Energy Healing* examines the state of our own physical energy field in relation to our total energy field, recommending that by looking after that energy field we can find the best path to a radiant, aligned, and positive physical energy. Crystals are wonderful energy tools for fulfilling this task.

There is no "dis-ease" of the physical that does not first begin in the energy field. Therefore, to treat our physical health a doctor may prescribe medication to help heal our physical body, but if we engage with crystal energy alongside a doctor's recommendations, our body will have the opportunity to heal faster. This is because we have engaged with our energy field by working with a crystal, a magnifier of positive energy. We have plugged into a huge, positive energy resource that can be programmed to meet the exact needs of our own energy field. What could be greater than that, and why aren't more of us waking up to this universal gift? Likewise, if after, say, a heart operation, we surround ourselves with crystals, we have the energetic opportunity to heal in half the time. Engaging with crystals can support the healing of broken bones, with energetic efforts also promoting healing time which, in turn, will be more flowing and faster. I have seen this take place over many years of working with crystals—it is not some form of miracle but rather is thanks to energy. Everything is energy. If we engage with the natural energy power source of crystals to align ourselves, our home, and our surroundings, the strengthened energy field will lead to a reduced chance of succumbing to, for example, Covid (see page 142).

Crystal Body Grids delivers the energy blueprint needed for forging a new way of living, going forward while learning from the past, empowering ourselves toward an energetically aware, Light-filled future. It helps us to realize that we are not just physical entities, but instead multidimensional beings and, as such, are tasked to wake up to our soul potential and realize this in an energy-harmonized and flowing body. It is my vision that the crystal energy healing configurations (or layouts/grids, depending on preferred terminology) outlined in each section of this book can form a framework for the reader to format with confidence their own personal crystal healing configurations that will meet their individual requirements for the well-being challenges we all face on a daily basis, as well as the energy enhancements we all seek. On that basis, the crystal healing configurations are not exhaustive, but rather a carefully chosen selection from the many configurations with which I have engaged in my nearly thirty years as a holistic therapist. It is my fervent hope that everyone will begin to engage naturally with crystals in order to support their "whole" being (holism for the whole energetic being) since we are, each of us, but energy. Treating ourselves, alongside physical medicine, with energetic antidotes seems a "no-brainer" to me on the basis that we are multidimensional beings, our physical "suit" being only one part of the great, big, whole energy being of each of us. We can claim the empowerment to enhance our life with the aligned forces of mind, body, and spirit simply by picking up a crystal. With this book at your side and your crystals at the ready, crystal energy can help you to achieve Light-filled, energy-enhanced health and well-being.

I wish you well on your journey,

Sharon L. McAllister

Part I

Crystal Healing

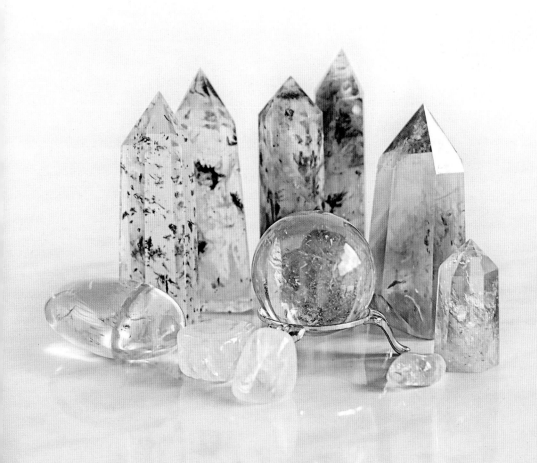

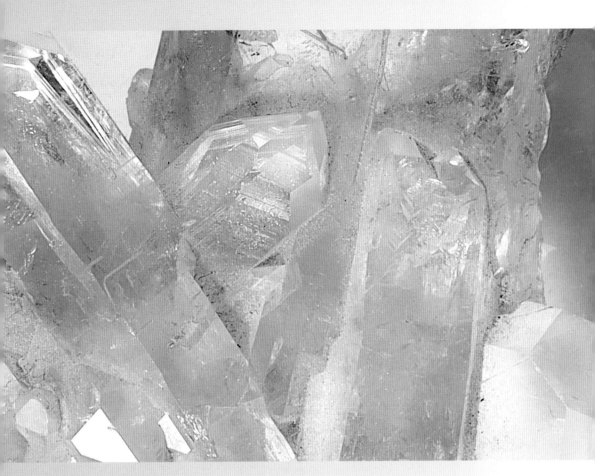

Chapter 1

Understanding Crystals and Energy

What is a crystal?

A crystal is a physical manifestation of Light energy. A pure quartz crystal is a myriad of vibrations of Light with many healing qualities. A rose quartz, for example, carries a specific vibration of Light, made physical, to embody and emit the Light of peace, healing, and unconditional love. Crystals are Light beings, just like us.

What is crystal healing?

Crystal healing is the application of crystals to the body and/or the chakras, and/or the placement of crystals at key points in the energy field of the person being treated. Crystals are manifestations of Light, and when they are "asked/programmed," they are charged with a magnification of Light energy that has the capacity to absorb negative energy in and around the body, while charging the energy within and around the body with enhancing Light energy. The Light energy seeks to balance, harmonize, and positivize the energy bodies of the person receiving crystal healing. Likewise, the crystals perform the same transmutative and positive energy charge when directed at other tasks, for example: aligning mind, body, and spirit in your children; raising the positive energy flow in your home or workplace; and healing negative places or the Earth's "sores." The list of applications where crystal healing can improve our lives is endless.

What is energy?

Energy is everything. You are energy planted into a physical body, and you use and apply that energy in a certain way. It is the same for a crystal: it is energy planted in a physical body and, like you, the universe has given each crystal a unique job. You give off energy. If your photograph were taken using Kirlian photography, for example, you would see a basic and somewhat crude interpretation of your energy in that particular moment. Yet your energy fluctuates all the time, nanosecond by nanosecond, with every thought, word, and deed, along with all the surrounding energy of people and places with which it comes into contact. The crystal has energy that pulses and radiates Light around it, and at the same time it also has the capacity to absorb negative energy.

Preparing yourself to use crystals: aligning your energy

Since crystals are such a powerful tool for increasing positive energy, a good way of preparing to be around and work with the energy of crystals is to align your own energy. By alignment I mean you should cleanse, clear, focus, and protect your energy field. The following method is effective for daily use, for example, before going out into the world each day. You will discover, and experience, that if you are *aligned*, your day will flow better and your energy levels will allow you to cope better with the energetic "stuff" that is thrown at you and with which everyone must deal. If you are experiencing a particularly challenging time, this process can be repeated at intervals throughout the day to help cleanse and charge your energy field.

Alignment of the self

- Stop your activities and be still.
- Call to the Light for energetic help: "I call on the Light (or earth energies), please help me at this time…"
- Breathe away the negativity from your body and your energy field by visualizing that you are breathing a beautiful blue Light from the crown of your head through the channel of your spine down to your feet, and away into the earth for transmutation.
- Breathe in the color emerald, a Light with a particularly high charge of positivity, and see this emerald Light wash from the crown of the head down through the body to the feet, grounding your

Light to the earth through your feet and through your arms and your hands.

- Seal yourself in a protective blue Light by visualizing a veil of blue Light energy above the crown of your head, extending out around your body to the tips of your fingers held at arm's length, and see this Light envelop you in an egg-like shape, sealing beneath your feet. Thank the Light (or earth energies).
- Be of joy and positivity.

It is also beneficial for positive energy to align your space (whether your home, room, workspace, or other environment) before working with crystals.

Alignment of your room

- Stop your activities and be still.
- Call for energetic help to cleanse yourself and your space: "I call to the Light (or earth energies). Please cleanse this room, all objects of this room, and myself of all negative energy. Please release this negative energy to the earth for transmutation. I thank the Light (or earth energies)."
- Call for energetic help to "positivize" yourself and your space: "I call on the Light (or earth energies). Please envelop this room, all objects of this room, and myself with the highest positivity for the energy required at this time (or the energy required of this day…). I thank the Light (or earth energies)."

I like to call the positive energetic action of cleansing yourself and your space, using the above alignment techniques *before* and *after* every healing session, together with that of cleansing your crystals (again both *before* and *after* every healing session), "good energy housekeeping."

Crystal care and cleansing

Why do we need to do this? Crystals require cleansing because they are powerful tools for the magnification and absorption of energy. Crystals that work hard on your behalf will have a containment point or limit. For example, if I dip a sponge into inky water, it will soak up the water and fill the sponge. Once filled to saturation point, the water that the sponge can no longer hold will start to drip back into the inky water, the saturation point of the sponge having been exceeded. Exactly the same happens with crystals. If you wear an amethyst for healing emotional energy, I feel sure that you would not wish to have that accumulated negative energy drip back into your energy field. Instead, I imagine you would want to release every drop of negativity, transmuting the negative feelings. Therefore, it is helpful to be energy-responsible and to cleanse the hard-working crystals accordingly.

How to cleanse your crystals

The amethyst bed

An amethyst bed is a natural piece of amethyst quartz crystal, in a reasonably flat, open shape upon which you can safely rest other crystals or your crystal jewelry. Ideally, an amethyst bed should be placed on or near a windowsill, or in sunlight (an energizing crystal cleansing vibration) for a minimum of three and a maximum of twelve hours. During this time, the sunlight works with the amethyst to cleanse and draw from the stone any held negative energy, absorbing and transmuting the latter. In the same way, moonlight energy cleansing transmutes challenging emotional holding from your crystals. To cleanse the amethyst bed, wash it in clean water and pat it dry before placing the amethyst in natural light once more to replenish its natural charge of energy.

The hands-on cleansing method

- Align yourself and your space.
- Place the crystals on a natural fiber cloth on a table in front of you.
- Call on the Light to cleanse the crystals: "I call on the Light (or earth energies). Please cleanse these crystals of all negative energy and release the negative energy from these crystals to the earth for transmutation."
- As you do so, rub your palm chakras together (to ignite their energy), sweep your palms three times over the crystals, and then sweep the negative energy "cloud" in a downward direction, literally dropping the energy from your hands, by your sides, to the earth. Then sweep your palms three times to the earth, releasing from them any residue of negativity. Ask for the earth to receive the negative energy for transmutation and thank the earth: "I thank the earth for transmuting this negative energy at this time."
- Call on the Light to recharge the crystals to the highest positivity: "I call on the Light (or earth energies). Please charge these crystals that they may be aligned to the highest positivity. I thank the Light."

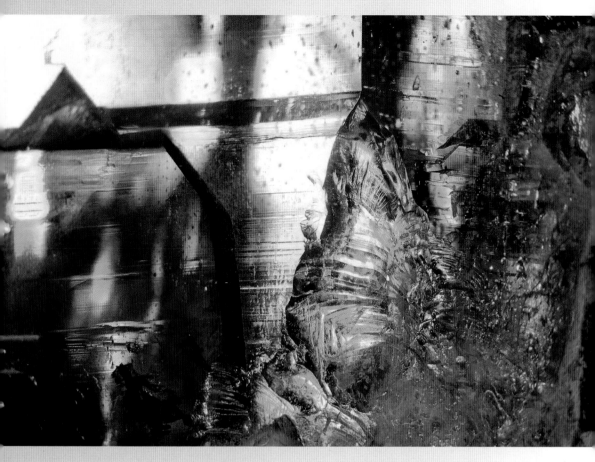

Chapter 2

Programming
Crystals for
Energy Healing

Simply asking your crystal is a form of programming. If you ask your crystal while holding it in the palm of your right hand, it will respond to your request only as long as your request is positive and within the crystal's energy remit. Think of this analogy: I could ask you to install my sink. That is fine if you are a plumber, but if you are not, you might make an attempt, but how effective would you be? A crystal always works best and most efficiently in the area of its universal remit (see the A–Z of Crystals on page 169 for a quick reference to the key qualities of crystals, along with suggestions on ways to apply their energy). A crystal will always work with a higher degree of energy amplification if asked/programmed to do so. If a crystal is never programmed, it is still working, but at its lowest volume. When you ask/program the crystal, it is charged, ready to ignite its full power and apply its energy to the task in hand. You have magnified its energetic Light charge many times over.

Let's say you have a rose quartz pendant and want to ask/program it to envelop you with the energy of peace when you wear it. Hold the pendant in the palm of your right hand and say: "I ask the Light (or earth energy if you prefer) that this rose quartz envelops me with the Light of peace. I thank the Light."

You may well think while reading this: Just a minute, I'm holding a rock in my hand and asking it to surround me with the energy of peace? How does that work? It sounds fantastical and it is. Energy is beyond amazing, but many of us have forgotten that everything is energy. We have forgotten that *we* are energy. A great number of us believe that we are merely physical matter moving about on the planet, yet in truth we are so much more. In reality, we are bright Lights of truly amazing energy, inhabiting a physical body, just as a crystal is an equally truly amazing energy in a rock or stone body.

Who exactly are you asking when you ask to charge/program a crystal? You are making an invocation to the Light/universe/earth energy, whichever higher power you are most comfortable with.

The energetic phenomenon is at the point at which you program a crystal and your energy meets the crystal energy (now resting on the palm of your hand) and something incredibly important happens. Your energy "puts its feelers out." In truth, your energy always has its feelers at the ready. Think about somewhere you have been that did not "feel" right. That is your intuition at work, your energy with its feelers out, constantly sensing and assessing the energy around you, even if you are not actually paying very much attention to this energetic messaging. Our energy field (our four lower bodies) is responding to the energy it meets all the time—retracting, expanding, shuddering, depleting—whether or not we are conscious of the positive or negative energy around us. Whether or not we like the idea, we are simply entirely made up of energy (vibrating at different rates) and need to learn to take care of our own energy by keeping our own energy fields in the most positive, Light-aligned, healthy, and vibrant flow that we can possibly muster.

Asking is a vibrational call. Energy follows thought, word, and deed. Therefore, in your act of asking, a pattern of vibrational energy meets the energy of the crystal and "patterns" it to what is required. It is like computer coding. You ask, and in so doing you are coding for a crystal. The crystal patterns to its vibrational requirement, just as you have asked it to do, therefore releasing the crystal's "tuning fork" capacity. The crystal then strikes the required vibrational note, depending on its remit (for example, rose quartz = the vibration of peace), and immediately the crystal's energy meets your own. The crystal then begins to hum its vibration of energy through and around you, with your energy drinking in the crystal's energy, sensing the charge of positivity, and facilitating the absorption of negative energy away from your own energy field into the crystal, together with the simultaneous charge of harmonizing balance. This particular energy will help you to feel cleaner and clearer, even if you have no cognitive awareness that this is happening.

When you ask/program the crystal, you are calling on the Light (or universe or earth energy, if you prefer) to charge the crystal with the "empowerment of Light," thus asking the crystal to be ignited for a particular positive purpose. The Light wants to positivize your energy and also that of our beautiful planet Earth. All we have to do is ask.

How do crystals work?

Crystals, like all natural gifts from the universe (from the earth energy, from the divine Light), are given to us to enhance and promote our positivity. The divine universe has blessed us with all we require to eat and drink, the need for shelter, and to have peace and love for each other, yet over time we human inhabitants of the Earth have successfully abused these gifts, collectively and individually. Crystals are a cosmic gift to us to boost our healing potential, to promote our connection to Spirit so that we may take responsibility and transmute our negative energy. Crystals perform this remarkable task by showing and reminding us of positive energy, giving us a model of that positive energy to follow in the pure vibration of Light. Our own energy recognizes this and, knowing inherently what its true positive state should be, follows the model energy state of the crystal. So, for example, when your heart is closed and has forgotten how to open, try wearing a rose quartz over your heart chakra. This crystal will vibrate its energy at a rate that reveals your depleted heart chakra: "This is how you can be. This is the beauty you can reveal, this is the way, this is the love, true and pure, that you can give. Follow my example." Like a tuning fork striking a musical note to follow, the molecular resonance of the crystal vibrates in order to show the imbalance within you the absolute equal and opposite positive energy for the negative, dis-eased part of your energy field to follow. The crystal strikes a vibration of pure energy, like the tuning fork and says: "Follow this note, follow this vibration of energy." Your energy, perhaps wobbly at first, perhaps in need of a number of sessions, begins to emulate the energetic vibrational note shown by the crystal. The crystal shows you the perfect mirror of pure energy vibration for your body and your energy field to become.

Crystal configurations, layouts, and circuits

A crystal configuration is a recipe-like layout of crystal energy. Its pattern (or grid) is made up of the alchemical conjunction of each individual crystal's energy, brought together as a whole in a vibrational pattern of Light energy that has the capacity to absorb any negative energy related to a particular energy challenge and bring a Light charge of positivity to, for example, a particular area of the body, as and when required.

Each energy challenge featured in the book is accompanied by a crystal configuration that provides a recipe (grid/layout) for the energetic placement of crystals for the tabletop (to sit before), the floor (to sit or lie on), or on and/or around the body. There are notes and tips on how best to apply this energetic healing as appropriate. Usually, a crystal configuration placed on the body as a layout works down from above the crown of the head, with crystals placed on chakra points and/or points where there is challenge or discomfort for the body, and so on, down to the feet. Crystals are sometimes mapped for placement at certain points away from the body, out in the energy field, where greater fine-tuning of the body's energy field can occur during the sessions.

The ignitor and exit crystals

In a crystal circuit the ignitor crystal is the charge, and the exit crystal the absorber. The ignitor brings pure Light energy to cleanse and positivize the energy field, while the exit crystal facilitates energetic transmutation of held negative energy. Switching on the energy charge to create a crystal circuit requires this ignitor crystal, which is usually a clear quartz tabular crystal with a shaped, pointed end. It should be directed toward the crown of the head and does not need to be large in size. It is partnered by an exit crystal, usually a single-terminated smoky quartz crystal with a point at one end, which is directed away from the body. The ignitor crystal forms the positive charge to the energy circuit, while the task of the exit crystal is to absorb the flow of negative energy that is released as the Light energy charges down from the ignitor crystal, through the body, through the energy field of the person undergoing crystal energy healing. The exit crystal acts as a kind of crystal vacuum cleaner, attracting and absorbing the negative energy flushed up and out into the energy field during the expansion of the four lower bodies that occurs during the crystal energy session.

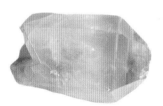

Fig. 1. Ignitor crystal

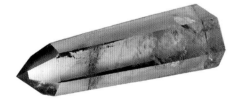

Fig. 2. Exit crystal

The Crystal Healing Session

How to create, open, ignite, and close the crystal circuit

You are ready to start. You have cleansed and aligned your energy, the energy of the room, and the energy of the crystals you wish to use. For help with placing the crystals correctly for each energy challenge, please refer to the body maps and the placement grids (layouts) shown in the diagrams. Without the ignitor/charge crystal, or the exit/absorber crystal, a grid is simply a grid, powerful though that may be. To create a circuit, to Light-charge and empower your grid, you will need an ignitor crystal, crystals that are to be positioned on and around the body, and the all-important exit crystal. Before positioning crystals on the body, place all the required crystals on the table, mapping them head to toe as shown in the diagram. Once you have checked that all the necessary crystals are present, you are ready to **ask/program these crystals** for the energetic healing session you require. You will find the relevant crystal program under the appropriate heading (see the example below).

Program the crystals for **crystals and chakra balancing** by asking:
    "I ask the Light (or earth energies), please charge these crystals with the highest positive energy to align, harmonize, and balance the chakra system of (full name). I thank the Light."

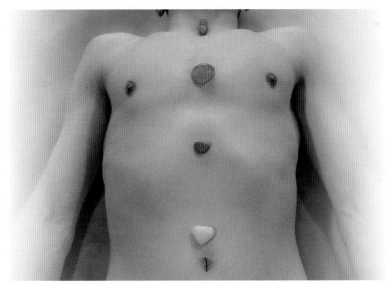

Crystals & chakra balancing

Fig 3. The chakra system

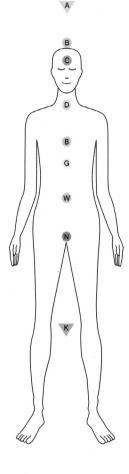

A = ignitor crystal
      clear quartz   12 inches (30 cm) above the crown chakra

B = rose quartz   1 inch (2.5 cm) above the crown chakra

C = lapis lazuli   third eye chakra

D = turquoise   throat chakra

B = rose quartz   heart chakra

G = rhodochrosite   solar plexus chakra

W = snow quartz   sacral chakra

N = ruby   base chakra

K = exit crystal
      smoky quartz   between the knees

Crystal energy healing time: 10 minutes
Aftercare: rest, drink water, and (if time allows) bathe or shower
Repeat session: weekly as required.

When your programmed crystals are ready, take your time and place the crystals on and around the body. Once the crystals are in position, a crystal circuit is created, which you are now ready to *ignite*.

To ignite the crystals, use a hands-on method. Place your palms together and twist them to ignite your own palm chakras, before placing your right hand about 6 inches (15 cm) above the heart chakra of the person receiving crystal energy healing, and ask:

"I call on the Light (or earth energies, if you prefer), please ignite the energy of these crystals to energy heal (full name) at this time. I thank the Light (or earth energies)."

Gently move the energy by rotating the palm of your hand over the heart chakra in a clockwise direction three times. Gently, and in a flowing movement, sweep your right hand, still at a level of 6 inches (15 cm) above the body, toward the exit crystal. Do this three times.

Time the session, which would usually be 10 minutes.

Close the crystal healing session by asking:

"I call on the Light (or earth energies), please close the energy of the crystals at this time. I thank the Light (or earth energies)."

Taking your time, with a flowing movement remove the crystals.

How to apply crystals on and around the body and remove them again

Everything is energy. The human energy field is made up of many bands, but for the purposes of the crystal energy healing grids in this book, we need to look at the four bands of energy that make up the four lower bodies of the human energy field located around the body. Nearest to the body is the physical energy band, which is roughly 3 to 6 inches (8 to 15 cm) above and around the whole body. The emotional energy band layered over the physical energy band is a further 6 inches (15 cm) beyond, and the mental energy band another 9 inches (23 cm) beyond the emotional energy band. Lastly, the spiritual energy band sits a further 12 inches (30 cm) out beyond the mental energy band. The four lower bodies usually complete at around an arm's length away from the body.

The crystal placement maps for each dis-ease of energy included in this book illustrate how to position the relevant crystals on and around the body. I usually place the ignitor and exit crystals first (following the requirements of the relevant crystal placement) in order to form the crystal circuit. I choose to do so because the person receiving crystal energy healing receives an instant pure charge of energy. From the ignitor crystal, Light energy pours through the body and the energy field, down through to the exit crystal at the knees or below the feet. Once the ignitor and exit crystal are in position, I place the crystals on the body, as mapped, beginning at the head and then working in a flowing movement down the body. If crystals are to be placed around the body, I usually work clockwise from the head around the body. Larger crystal configurations requiring crystals to be placed beyond the body are often best carried out on a large bed or on (or around) a blanket or yoga mat on the floor.

When it is time to remove the crystals, I collect them from around the body first, using a flowing movement, and then gently and slowly remove the crystals from the body itself (remember the energy field/chakras can be very sensitive for some people). Finally, I remove the ignitor crystal and then the exit crystal, leaving the latter to the very end since it will continue to absorb the residue of energy released into the energy field despite the energy of the crystals having been "closed" prior to removing them. Be assured that your energy field will be clearer and charged with positive energy following the session. Be aware too that the effects of crystal energy healing continue to work for up to twenty-four hours after a session. Crystals can also be carried or worn between sessions. However, crystal energy healing is a deep healing, and is usually carried out at weekly or monthly intervals, often interspersed with other body therapies, such as holistic reflexology or aromatherapy massage, which keep your energy field moving and flowing. Crystal energy healing has the potential to absorb your negative energy and charge up your energy field to a far greater degree than most other therapies. Recommended optimum time frames for repeat sessions of the various crystal energy healing treatments are included with the diagrams.

Cleanse your crystals in cold water, or use the hands-on energy cleansing method (see page 18).

Aftercare

Crystal energy healing is powerful and the person who has received it may feel rather "spaced out" following the sessions. This is because the energy field expands several feet beyond the point at which it naturally sits at arm's length from the body. It is a good idea to drink water, rest, and have a light meal or snack, requiring the physical body to function by processing the food and liquid, thereby pulling the energy field back to its natural, resident state. It is no longer out in the room, but back within arm's length of the body. It is also helpful to bathe or take a shower after a crystal healing session. Do not drive until you feel fully awake and aware.

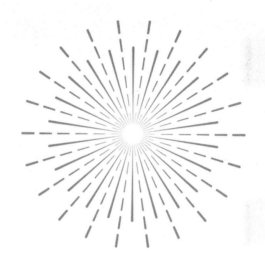

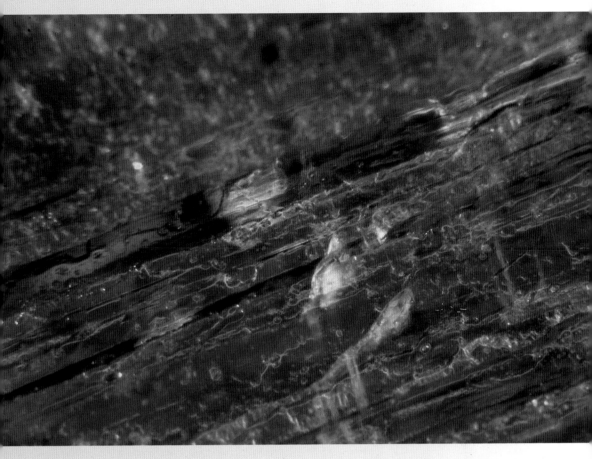

Chapter 3

The Human Energy Field, Chakras, and the Metaphysics of Dis-ease

The chakra system

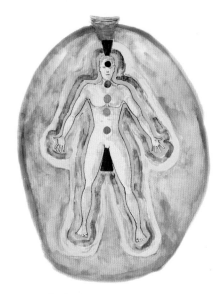

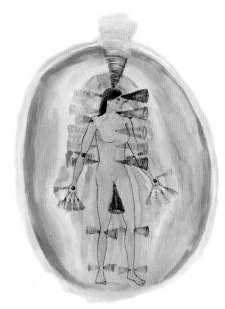

Fig. 4. The human energy field, the chakra system (7 major chakras)

Fig. 5. The human energy field, the wider chakra system (52 major and minor chakras)

There is no dis-ease of the physical body that does not first begin in the energy field. We may find this hard to believe, but that is because most of us have forgotten that we even have an energy field, and yet our very physical health depends, first and foremost, on the care and health of our personal energy field.

Are you breathing?

Take a moment to sit with your eyes closed and become aware of your lungs moving in and out as they receive and expel air. You need this air to breathe and, amazingly enough, your body converts this energy, this air, gathering in the oxygen you require and expelling the carbon dioxide you no longer need. This process, known as gas exchange, is essential to life.

Most people believe that this energy, together with food and drink, is all the physical nourishment they require, but human bodies are far more complex than that. Positive energy that feeds the human energy field is as important as air and physical food or drink.

So, what is this energy and where does it come from?

Energy is the universal Light emitted from the Source, the Godhead. It is as real and tangible as any physical object you can see and touch. It is the very stuff of life. Without this energy nourishment we cannot function, and the way that we take in this energy is through our chakra system. The chakra system is just as important to us as, say, the respiratory system.

Therefore, I repeat the question: Are you breathing? With your lungs perhaps, but are you breathing with your energy system? Asking ourselves how healthy our lungs are is not something we often take time to do, since breathing is automatic and most of us do not have to think about it unless we have dis-ease or live in a polluted atmosphere, for example. Asking ourselves how healthy our chakras are is also something the majority of people on this planet currently do not often stop and do. Why is that?

More often it is a lack of energy awareness, a refusal to acknowledge the energy bodies, and/or a denial of their Light connection that leads to failure by a great many of us to focus on the health of our energy fields. The manifestation of this lack of awareness cannot be ignored, as was the case when smokers began to partake, globally, in polluting their lungs, and vast increases in disease (lung, heart, vascular . . .) occurred en masse. Smokers once had a lack of awareness, but we now know that smoking causes negativity that pollutes our bodies, resulting in disease and premature death in some cases. When it comes to denial of the human energy field, as energy field workers with an understanding of the human energy system, we know that lack of awareness can result in a dis-eased and uncared for energy system, leading to damaged, torn, blocked, leaking, ruptured, and even closed chakras.

Take a moment to pause and consider your own chakra system.

How many of your own chakras do you "feel" are open, fully flowing, fully working?

All? Some? Or none?

It may surprise you to know that it is more likely to be none. If you are committed to a lifelong healing and meditation program, you are probably better off in the sense that your chakra system will have more flow. If you feel you have a fully open and flowing chakra system, you may need to think again; we live in difficult times, with many energy challenges constantly pressuring our four lower bodies, so we would have to work very hard to achieve a total, fully flowing energy system for much of our life. This is why it is best to work through a personal healing program to check in with the health of our energy fields, together with keeping our energy cleansed and maintaining our positive energy levels.

In reality, it is most likely that you will have some *open* chakras, but which are not yet energy cleansed or as flowing in positive energy as

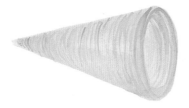

Fig. 6. A healthy chakra (single vortex)

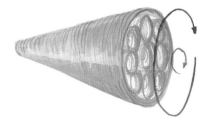

Fig. 7. A healthy chakra (multivortex)

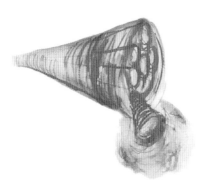

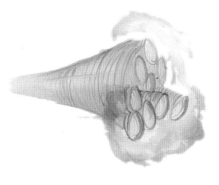

Fig. 8. The beginning of a dis-eased chakra (sacral chakra)

Fig. 9. The broken heart chakra

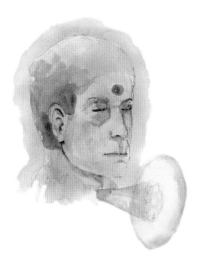

Fig. 10. A closed chakra (third eye) and an armored chakra (throat)

they might be, and some *damaged* chakras. Look at any dis-eases or physical ailments you are experiencing or to which may be suscepti-ble—the clues to the chakras on which you need to work will be there. Your body reveals where you have energy flow blocks. You will also have some *closed* chakras. Over 95 percent of the Earth's population has a closed base chakra. If you have the latter, there is a major bung in your personal energy plumbing.

The Threefold Energy System Charge

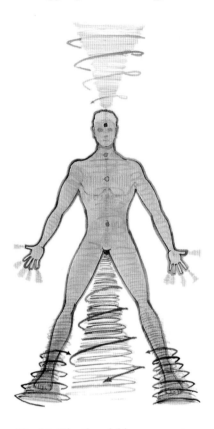

Fig. 11. The threefold energy system
This image shows primary energy coming down through the crown chakra,
earth energy coming up through the feet, and universal energy being drawn
in by the chakra system.

Primary energy flow moves through the crown of the head, down through the spine, and grounds to the earth. Earth energy moves through the "minor" chakras in the feet and rises up through the body. Each of these energies flow, fountain-like, in the body, through and around it.

Just like the lungs, the chakra system draws the universal energy in and out: positive energy in, with the release of karmic residue out. It is similar to the respiratory system, which mirrors this energy system.

There is **the threefold energy system charge**.

Primary energy: pure Light divine connection.

Universal energy: positive energy.

Earth energy: your connection to earth, your grounding energy to allow you to release your karmic energy.

Karmic energy

Karmic energy is both positive and negative. When we begin our journey from birth it is neutral. It is our task throughout life to build up positive energy, but life brings many opportunities, good and bad, and sometimes we make decisions that create negative energy. It is then our task to positivize this negative energy, creating positive karma, with a hope that, when we come to the end of our existence, we have created more positive than negative karma, or at least neutralized all that negative energy in our lives.

Using crystals to positivize negative blocks helps to release negative energy and positivize the energy around our body in order to prevent negative karma building up in our energy field.

Think of a cake divided into each day of your life that you will eat, and your body will process and release, as with any food. Processing karma is similar, and some days you may ask for a larger slice of cake and on others a smaller one. For some people the cake slices may be piling up because they are not processing the karmic residue as they requested to do prior to entering this life. For cake, read any of life's struggles and challenges: illness, lack of patience, loss, overcoming adversity, giving, sharing, anger, bitterness, and so on.

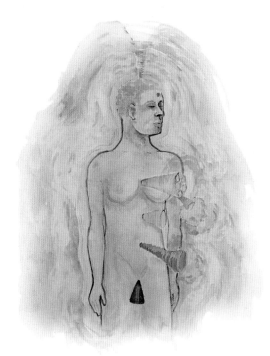

Fig. 12. A typical human energy field.
This image shows a closed third eye and throat chakra, a heart chakra
in emotional crisis, a weak solar plexus chakra, a sacral chakra that is
"blowing off" negative energy in a process of emotional turmoil, and
a base chakra that is shorter, not fully functioning because it is
on its way to becoming blocked.

How do crystals help us with all this energy that we have to process?

Crystals have the capacity to *absorb* negative energy, with some crystals resonant to work specifically in harmony with certain parts of the body and/or certain forms of energy dis-ease. Crystals also have the capacity to *charge* our bodies and our energy fields with positive energy, a pure high charge of energy to replenish and heal where negativity has been released.

If you change just one thing: the energy of kyanite

Kyanite is a master crystal. A master crystal has properties that elevate its inherent qualities. This is a substantial topic in itself, but for the purposes of this example it is enough to know that kyanite has the capacity to self-cleanse—to transmute the negative energy it has drawn in and realign its natural high charge positive state without the requirement for the user/therapist to energy cleanse or place it in water, and so on. I would still recommend including kyanite when cleansing crystals. Kyanite has the capacity to align and physically strengthen the wearer or carrier, and it is a powerful crystal with which to work when programmed. For example, cleanse and program a kyanite like this:

> "I call upon the Light (or the earth energies), please program this crystal to energy align and strengthen me (or full name) in my daily life. I thank the Light (or earth energies)."

When you first start to wear kyanite, you may experience the feeling of having just had your "electrics switched on." You may have been feeling tired and lethargic, perhaps with a dullness in terms of general energy levels. Kyanite engenders a feeling of positivity, of realignment. I have known energy skeptics who have begun wearing kyanite, experienced a shift in their sense of positivity, questioned this (how can it possibly be from a crystal?), removed the kyanite, and then felt, almost immediately, a drop in their positive energy. Once they wore the kyanite again, they noticed an uplift in strengthened energy, a feeling that they could move through any challenges they were facing, with an empowered "I can do this" energy moving forward.

If we could all "see" the energy field like an energy intuitive (who has the gift to see the human energy field), we would observe that when wearing kyanite, the wearer's energy is constantly regenerating, their chakras are open, and they are standing straighter and stronger than before wearing the crystal. Their energy field looks much healthier. It would be clear to the energy intuitive that the kyanite had enhanced the flow of energy in the field, helping to clear and align the meridians and chakras, in turn allowing the negative energy to exit the energy circuit. The kyanite does not set up the circuit (that is your own energy field), but rather the kyanite's programming encourages alignment by effecting a positive change of energy, using all your energy field's positive attributes to enable this process. This can be likened to an amplifier on a music system: the system still works without the amplifier, but not as well. With kyanite as the amplifier, your energetic vibration is fine-tuned and the volume turned up.

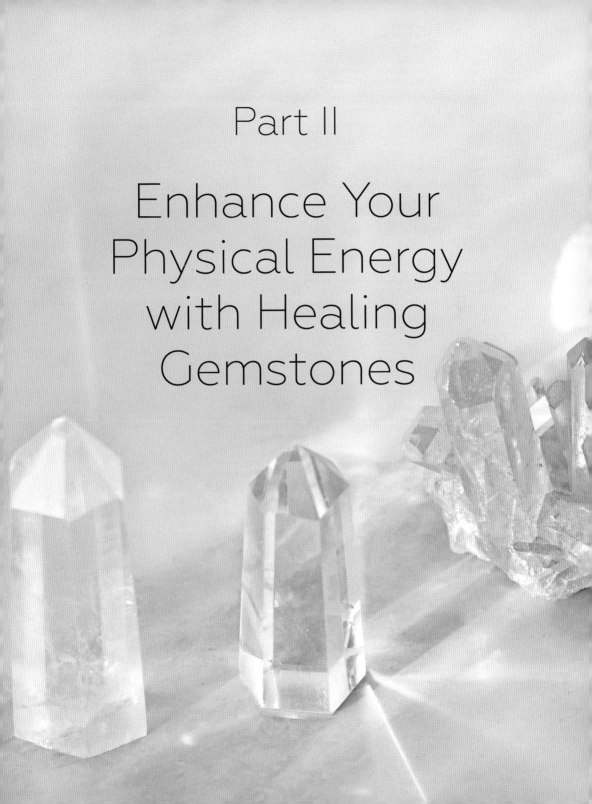

Part II

Enhance Your Physical Energy with Healing Gemstones

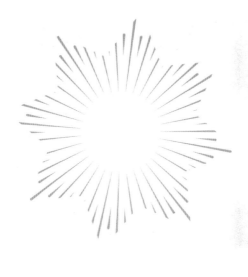

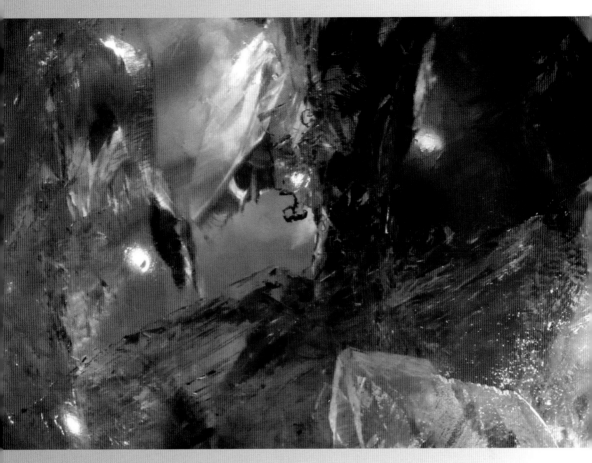

The Skeletal Structure, Nerves, and Pain

Energetic pain relief

The energy example we will look at here focuses on nerve pain in males in the groin from a back injury, where the pain extends around the stomach (causing spasms) and travels down into the rectum, penis, and testicles. The grid shown here would work on anyone experiencing stomach spasms and groin discomfort. (There is no gender bias in the layouts included in this book.) Pink calcite bars or rose mangano bars have the energetic resonance to meet the biting energy of nerve pain. Clients with whom I have worked who suffer with this type of difficulty describe how calcite or mangano bars "take the edge off" the intense pain, which is very helpful when this is so debilitating. These crystals can be programmed and held by the person experiencing the extreme pain, or they can be placed under a pillow to help make rest or sleep with such pain easier. They can be used in conjunction with a crystal configuration, as shown in the diagram opposite. Program the crystals by asking:

"I call upon the Light (or the earth energies), please charge these crystals to bring energetic pain relief to (full name) at this time. I thank the Light."

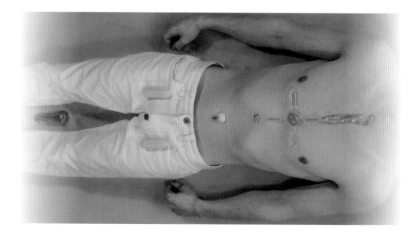

Fig 13. Energetic pain relief

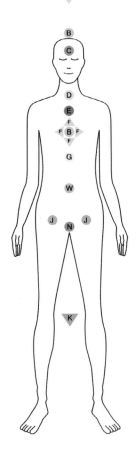

A =	ignitor crystal	12 inches (30 cm) above the crown chakra
B =	rose quartz	1 inch (2.5 cm) above the crown chakra
C =	lapis lazuli	third eye chakra
D =	turquoise	throat chakra
E =	blue kyanite	thymus (halfway between the throat and heart chakras)
B =	rose quartz	heart chakra
F =	4 clear quartz	single-terminated, directed outward around the rose quartz
G =	rhodochrosite	solar plexus chakra
W =	snow quartz	sacral chakra
J =	2 rose mangano	placed on the areas of greatest pain
N =	ruby	base chakra
K =	exit crystal	between the knees

Crystal energy healing time: 10 minutes
Aftercare: rest, drink water, and (if time allows) bathe or shower
Repeat session: twice a month
Notes: pink calcite or rose quartz can replace rose mangano crystals.

Energy strengthening the spine (weakness and injury)

We have a choice of two different crystals in this instance. Abalone is gentler and can be applied more regularly. Use it weekly for pain relief, gentle energy healing, to release held energy, or to regenerate a positive energy charge to the affected area. It can also be placed on a number of centers of injury. I used microporous tape to apply several abalone crystals to the plaster casts of a client who had suffered multiple fractures in a nasty motorbike accident. I have also placed it, for example, on a fractured collarbone.

Rutilated quartz crystal is more powerful and can cause clients some discomfort during the session since it disturbs the emotional energy held in the spine. Its use should be guided by the requirements of the individual and their level of comfort with this process; if they find it uncomfortable, use abalone instead.

The person to be treated with crystal energy healing can lie on their stomach on a bed, with abalone placed on their back or rutilated quartz crystal on the corresponding site of the back injury. Some people are not comfortable lying on their front or back, so work to suit the needs and comfort of the individual.

Program the crystals for **energy strengthening of the spine** by asking:

"*I ask the Light (or earth energies), please charge these crystals with the highest positive energy to envelop (full name) with the Light of transmutation, energetic healing, peace, and alignment that the framework of their life may be of greater strength. I thank the Light.*"

Fig 14. Energy strengthening the spine (weakness and injury)

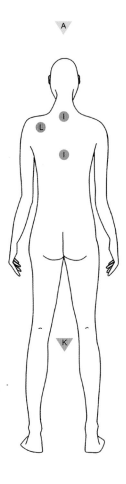

A = ignitor crystal   8 inches (20 cm) above the crown chakra

L = abalone   1 piece / multiple pieces on the site/s of pain/injury

OR

I = rutilated quartz crystal [Fred, take down 'crystal'?]

K = exit crystal   between the knees

Crystal energy healing time: 10 minutes
Aftercare: rest, drink water, and (if time allows) bathe or shower
Repeat session: weekly as required
Notes: the exit crystal may also be placed between the ankles (this turns down the volume on the energetic pull of the exit crystal).

Energy mending and strengthening bones (breaks and degeneration)

This crystal healing layout supports the energetic mending of bones that have undergone a fracture or some form of degeneration. This crystal layout example is used to strengthen energy in cases of weakness in the knees and breakage to the tibia (shin bone).

Program the crystals for **energy mending and strengthening bones** by asking:

'I ask the Light (or earth energies), please charge these crystals with the highest positive energy to envelop (full name) with the Light of transmutation, energetic healing, peace, strength, and alignment. I thank the Light."

Fig. 15. Energy mending and strengthening bones (breaks and degeneration)

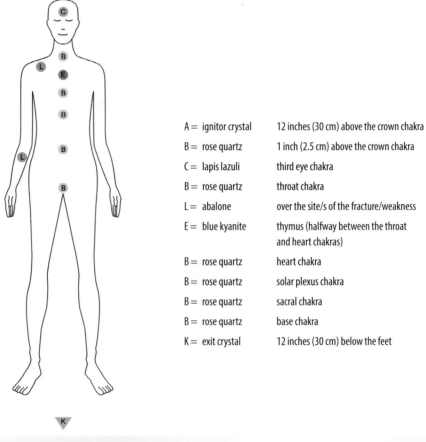

A =	ignitor crystal	12 inches (30 cm) above the crown chakra
B =	rose quartz	1 inch (2.5 cm) above the crown chakra
C =	lapis lazuli	third eye chakra
B =	rose quartz	throat chakra
L =	abalone	over the site/s of the fracture/weakness
E =	blue kyanite	thymus (halfway between the throat and heart chakras)
B =	rose quartz	heart chakra
B =	rose quartz	solar plexus chakra
B =	rose quartz	sacral chakra
B =	rose quartz	base chakra
K =	exit crystal	12 inches (30 cm) below the feet

Crystal energy healing time: 10 minutes
Aftercare: rest, drink water, and (if time allows) bathe or shower
Repeat session: weekly as required
Notes: use as many pieces of abalone as required, they can be secured in place with microporous tape.

Energy mending and strengthening hip bones (arthritis)

Citrines are powerful crystals for absorbing negative, stuck energy, for reducing energy blockages, and for general cleansing of the energy field. Citrine charges blocked areas with positive energy to stimulate greater flow and deliver balance in the energy field. For an energy blockage to the knee, for example, place a citrine crystal on the center of the painful area. Using microporous tape to secure a crystal in place helps both to position it correctly and to prevent it from rolling off during the healing session. You can, of course, also secure the crystal with tape over clothes. We are working with energy, which, if visible to the naked eye, would be billowing out around the knee, away from the body at some distance through the energy field.

Program the crystals for **energy mending and strengthening bones (arthritis)** by asking:

> "I ask the Light (or earth energies), please charge these crystals with the highest positive energy to envelop (full name) with the Light of transmutation, energetic healing, peace, strength, and alignment, so that they can move forward in empowerment. I thank the Light."

Fig. 16. Energy mending and strengthening hip bones (arthritis)

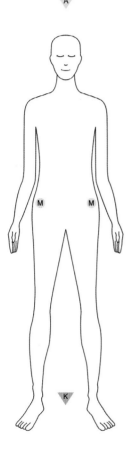

A = ignitor crystal   8 inches (20 cm) above the crown chakra

M = citrine   1 piece / multiple pieces on the site/s of pain/injury

K = exit crystal   between the ankles

Crystal energy healing time: 10 minutes
Aftercare: rest, drink water, and (if time allows) bathe or shower
Repeat session: weekly as required.

Energy mending and strengthening knee bones (arthritis)

Program the crystals for **energy mending and strengthening knee bones (arthritis)** by asking:

"I ask the Light (or earth energies), please charge these crystals with the highest positive energy to envelop (full name) with the Light of transmutation, energetic healing, peace, strength, and alignment, so that they can move forward in greater flexibility in life. I thank the Light."

Fig. 17. Energy mending and strengthening knee bones (arthritis)

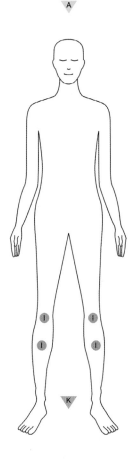

A = ignitor crystal   8 inches (20 cm) above the crown chakra

I = rutilated quartz   1 piece / multiple pieces on the site/s
of pain/injury

K = exit crystal   between the ankles

Crystal energy healing time: 10 minutes
Aftercare: rest, drink water, and (if time allows) bathe or shower
Repeat session: weekly as required.

Energy mending and strengthening hand bones (arthritis)

Sit comfortably and place the affected hand on a table beside you, setting out the crystals as indicated and using as many citrines as you require. Secure them in place directly over the painful or affected areas using microporous tape or similar.

Program the crystals for **energy mending and strengthening hand bones (arthritis)** by asking:

> "I ask the Light (or earth energies), please charge these crystals with the highest positive energy to envelop (full name) with the Light of transmutation, energetic healing, peace, strength, and alignment, so that they can move forward with greater empowerment in life. I thank the Light."

Fig. 18. Energy mending and strengthening hand bones (arthritis)

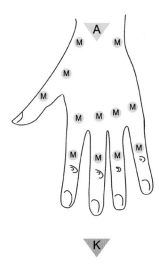

A = ignitor crystal   resting to a point above the wrist

M = citrines   1 piece / multiple pieces on the site/s of pain/injury

K = exit crystal   2 inches (5 cm) beyond the hand

Crystal energy healing time: 10 minutes
Aftercare: rest, drink water, and (if time allows) bathe or shower
Repeat session: weekly as required
Notes: with the hand placed flat on a table for the duration of the session, crystals can be secured on the hand and fingers with microporous tape.

The energy of cellular regeneration (general energy healing)

I recommend this particular crystal energy healing for a general pick-me-up. The energetic role of cellular regeneration is to physically realign, through crystals, the cellular structure of the body: cells, sinews, tissues, muscles, skeleton, and skin (in short, any dense physical matter).

The cellular regeneration crystal healing layout/grid can be used for the energy of general physical well-being, debilitation after illness or surgery, physical degeneration (such as through aging), or indeed physical wear and tear in those who play a lot of sport.

Program the crystals by asking:

"I call upon the Light (or the earth energies), please charge these crystals with the highest positivity to energetically regenerate the four lower bodies of (full name). I thank the Light."

Fig. 19. The energy of cellular regeneration (general energy healing) – 1

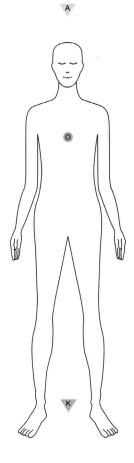

A = ignitor crystal   8 inches (20 cm) above the crown chakra

O = emerald   heart chakra

K = exit crystal   between the ankles

Crystal energy healing time: 10 minutes

Aftercare: rest, drink water, and (if time allows) bathe or shower

Repeat session: weekly as required

Notes: do not underestimate the power of this energy healing. After the session has been completed, many people report feeling as though they have been "plugged in" to a power source, with a greater feeling of physical alignment and clarity.

Fig. 20. The energy of cellular regeneration (general energy healing) – 2

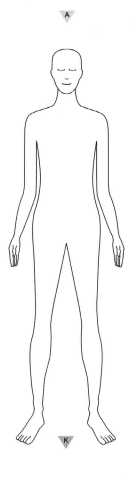

A = ignitor crystal   8 inches (20 cm) above the crown chakra

K = exit crystal   3 inches (8 cm) below the feet

Crystal energy healing time: 10 minutes
Aftercare: rest, drink water, and (if time allows) bathe or shower
Repeat session: weekly as required
Notes: this energy healing offers the opportunity to lie within a circuit of pure Light energy charge from the ignitor crystal while accumulated negative energy is transmuted by the pull of the exit crystal. The only way I can describe it is that it is like having an energetic shower – like a water shower – the effect is reviving, refreshing, and revitalizing.

Chapter 5

The Heart and
Vascular System

The energy of asthma*

Breathing is all about the positive flow of your energetic life force. To support the energy of peace, healing, and positive flow, use rose quartz and combine its energy with that of a rhodochrosite crystal. When treating children, begin by introducing a programmed crystal for them to wear or carry in a pouch secured inside or on a garment. Adults can start by wearing a programmed rose quartz crystal over the heart chakra, alternating it every two days with a programmed rhodochrosite crystal worn over the solar plexus chakra. If easier, the crystals can be carried in a pouch or pocket.

Program the crystals for **the energy of asthma** by asking:

"I ask the Light (or earth energies), please charge these crystals with the highest positive energy to veil (full name) with the energy of peace and the Light energy of healing to their respiratory system. I thank the Light."

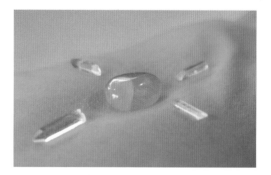

* For all health challenges, please seek advice from a physical doctor to go hand in hand with the energy therapy you undertake.

Fig. 21. The energy of asthma

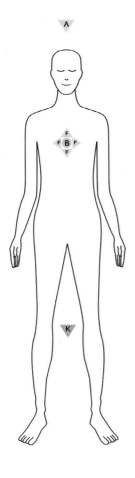

A = ignitor crystal   8 inches (20 cm) above the crown chakra

B = rose quartz   heart chakra

F = 4 clear quartz   single-terminated (directed outward) around the rose quartz

K = exit crystal   between the knees

Crystal energy healing time: 10 minutes
Aftercare: rest, drink water, and (if time allows) bathe or shower
Repeat session: every week for 3 weeks, followed by a month's gap, and then repeat for another 3 weeks, as required
Notes: older children can wear/carry a programmed rose quartz. For younger children, place a large programmed rose quartz centrally within the home, but out of the reach of small children, to allow a peaceful veil of energy to move in, through, and around.

The energy of heart dis-ease

The heart chakra has a primary function in the human energy field. We are designed by the Light to emit positive energy and receive Light energy in turn, and this exchange of energy flows and repeats throughout our lives. Our hearts are programmed by the Light before birth with an infinite capacity to love and give out a positive, loving, and free-flowing energy. We learn to shield, close, withdraw, withhold, and protect our heart energy from an early age in our physical life. Keeping our heart chakras healthy and flowing has the capacity to change, for the better, how we live and experience life and how we gift and benefit those around us and the wider world.

To align and start to heal your heart energy, begin by wearing or carrying a programmed rose quartz, alternating this each day with a programmed amethyst. These two crystals will work together in alchemical harmony to cleanse the energy field and the heart chakra, as well as strengthening the heart chakra and increasing positive flow to combat stagnation in the energy field. The length of time dedicated to wearing crystals depends on how the wearer feels. I recommend it as positive "homework" between crystal healing appointments, and it is an empowering thing to do for yourself. Most people feel a positive shift when wearing crystals and choose to continue to do so until they feel better. This may vary from a week to a month or more, depending on the wearer, who can then progress to a crystal layout/grid such as the one shown here.

Program the crystals for **the energy of heart dis-ease** by asking:

"I ask the Light (or earth energies), please charge these crystals with the highest positive energy to envelop (full name) with the Light to promote energetic heart chakra healing, peace, harmony, alignment, and flow. I thank the Light."

Fig. 22. The energy of the heart dis-ease

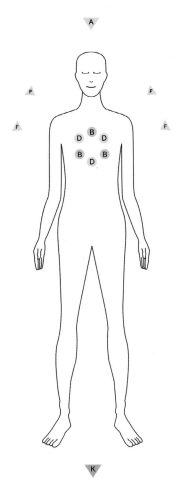

A = ignitor crystal	24 inches (60 cm) above the crown chakra
B = 3 rose quartz	at 12, 4 and 8 o'clock around the heart chakra
D = 3 turquoise	at 2, 6 and 10 o'clock around the heart chakra
F = 4 quartz crystal	single-terminated (8 inches/20 cm) beyond the body (directed toward the body)
K = exit crystal	8 inches (20 cm) below the feet

Crystal energy healing time: 10 minutes
Aftercare: rest, drink water, and (if time allows) bathe or shower
Repeat session: twice a month.

The energy of balancing blood pressure

Begin by wearing or carrying a programmed rose quartz, and then weave in weekly sessions of crystal therapy. A combination of ruby, kyanite, and rose quartz, together with a single-terminated clear quartz crystal, is included in this crystal layout.

Program the crystals for **the energy of balancing blood pressure** by asking:

> *"I ask the Light (or earth energies), please charge these crystals with the highest positive energy to envelop (full name) with the healing energy to bring peace, calm, and alignment to their condition, to energy balance blood pressure. I thank the Light."*

Fig. 23. The energy of balancing blood pressure

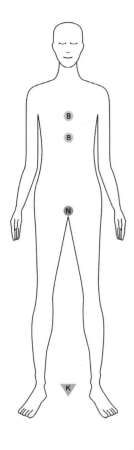

B = rose quartz   heart chakra

B = rose quartz   solar plexus chakra

N = ruby   base chakra

K = exit crystal   between the ankles

Crystal energy healing time: 10 minutes
Aftercare: rest, drink water, and (if time allows) bathe or shower
Repeat session: twice a month
Notes: there is **no** ignitor crystal for this layout/grid. The human energy field is gently cleansed and the chakras are brought into energy flow once more.

The energy of balancing blood sugar

Crystals provide a powerful natural support to any condition in which the body is out of balance and seeks to restore it. This applies even if medication has been prescribed by a medical practitioner. Crystals are noninvasive (they simply change energy), and crystal energy ignites positive change in the four lower bodies, where balance is always sought. (Always consult your doctor with any health condition you are experiencing.) Wearing or carrying kyanite programmed to balance the body and suppress the negative energy that needs or feeds on sugar is a good way to begin, before introducing a crystal configuration such as the one shown here.

Program the crystals for **the energy of balancing blood sugar** by asking:

> *"I ask the Light (or earth energies), please charge these crystals with the highest positive energy to envelop (full name) with the healing energy to bring peace, harmony, and alignment to their energy field to bring greater balance to their blood. I thank the Light."*

Fig. 24. The energy of balancing blood sugar

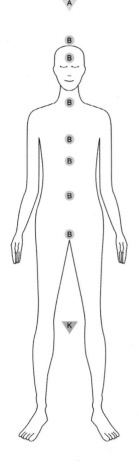

A =	ignitor crystal	12 inches (30 cm) above the crown chakra
B =	rose quartz	1 inch (2.5 cm) above the crown chakra
B =	rose quartz	third eye chakra
B =	rose quartz	throat chakra
B =	rose quartz	heart chakra
B =	rose quartz	solar plexus chakra
B =	rose quartz	sacral chakra
B =	rose quartz	base chakra
K =	exit crystal	between the knees

Crystal energy healing time: 10 minutes
Aftercare: rest, drink water, and (if time allows) bathe or shower
Repeat session: weekly as required.

The energy of purifying blood

Some people find it challenging to get on top of a physical infection. Those who have endured low level infection and have been on antibiotics for long periods, which in itself can cause many issues, are able to find energetic help by wearing or carrying hematite programmed to purify the blood. This is a good introduction to crystal use and helps to build a person's energy in preparation for placing crystal configurations on and around the body. If you are unable to find hematite, wear or carry an amethyst instead, and then move on to the crystal layout shown here.

Program the crystals for **the energy of purifying blood** by asking:

"I ask the Light (or earth energies), please charge these crystals with the highest positive energy to envelop (full name) with the healing energy to purify, align, and rebalance their blood. I thank the Light."

Fig. 25. The energy of purifying blood

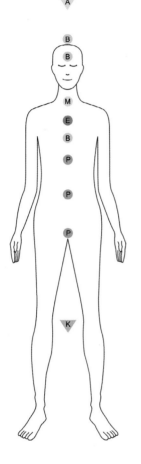

A =	ignitor crystal	12 inches (30 cm) above the crown chakra
B =	rose quartz	1 inch (2.5 cm) above the crown chakra
B =	rose quartz	third eye chakra
M =	citrine	throat chakra
E =	blue kyanite	thymus (halfway between the throat and heart chakras)
B =	rose quartz	heart chakra
P =	amethyst	solar plexus chakra
P =	amethyst	sacral chakra
P =	amethyst	base chakra
K =	exit crystal	between the knees

Crystal energy healing time: 10 minutes
Aftercare: rest, drink water, and (if time allows) bathe or shower
Repeat session: weekly as required.

The energy of varicose veins

The method outlined here can be used in conjunction with a crystal layout where the ignitor crystal is placed 12 inches (30 cm) above the head and the exit crystal is placed between the knees or 12 inches (30 cm) below the feet in order to establish the energy circuit. Alternatively, tape the programmed crystal onto the center of the affected area and wear it in bed.

Amethyst works well for energy blockages, whereas for visible thread veins I would choose a flat selenite crystal (a lightweight massage stone), and use microporous tape to secure it to the area as required. In my own experience, many clients find it helpful to apply this kind of crystal energy healing overnight.

Program the crystals for **the energy of varicose veins** by asking:

"I ask the Light (or earth energies), please charge these crystals with the highest positive energy to envelop (full name) with the Light of flowing harmony and energetic healing to their vascular system. I thank the Light."

Fig. 26. The energy of varicose veins

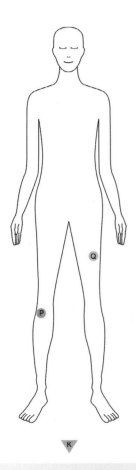

A = ignitor crystal   12 inches (30 cm) above the crown chakra

P = amethyst   directly onto the varicose veins

K = exit crystal   12 inches (30 cm) below the feet

OR

A = ignitor crystal   12 inches (30 cm) above the crown chakra

Q = selenite   directly onto the thread veins

K = exit crystal   12 inches (30 cm) below the feet

OR

Combine both of the above layouts as shown

Crystal energy healing time: 10 minutes

Aftercare: rest, drink water, and (if time allows) bathe or shower

Repeat session: weekly as required

Notes: choose lightweight massage stone selenite or lightweight bars. The amethyst/selenite can be carefully secured with microporous tape.

The energy of edema

A localized edema occurring, for example, in your left leg, perhaps in and around the ankle, can be helped energetically by using a programmed fluorite. A small fluorite crystal would be suitable, or a flat massage stone. Use microporous tape to apply it to the center of the affected site as shown, and also tape it into position at night in order for it to work on your behalf while you sleep. Wearing or carrying a fluorite or peridot helps to get the energy field moving as well as to reduce any stagnant energy sitting in the energy field. A fluorite crystal applied with tape can be used in conjunction with a crystal energy healing configuration, as shown. This can also be set up in a crystal circuit, with both an ignitor and exit crystal to turn up the volume on the energetic pull.

Program the crystals for **the energy of edema** by asking:

"I ask the Light (or earth energies), please charge these crystals with the highest positive energy to envelop (full name) with the Light of flowing harmony, energetic healing, balance, and alignment at this time. I thank the Light."

Fig. 27. The energy of edema

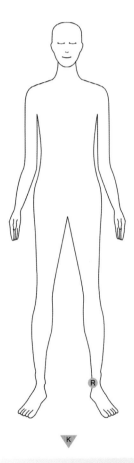

A = ignitor crystal   12 inches (30 cm) above the crown chakra

R = fluorite crystal   center of where the energy block is located

K = exit crystal   12 inches (30 cm) below the feet

Crystal energy healing time: 10 minutes
Aftercare: rest, drink water, and (if time allows) bathe or shower
Repeat session: weekly as required.

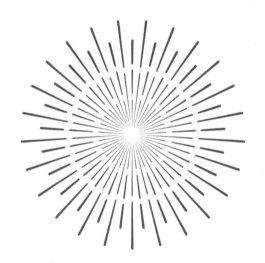

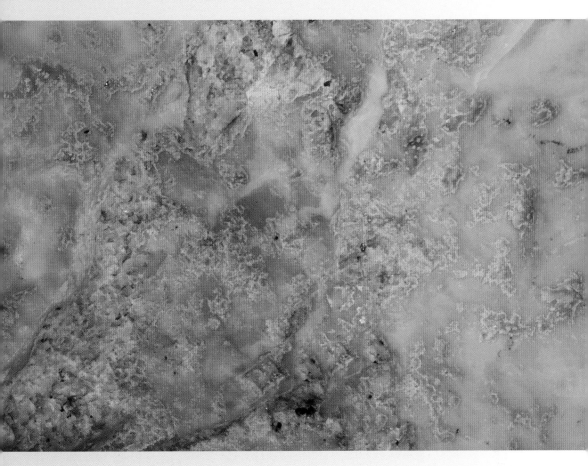

Chapter 6

The Gut and Digestion

The energy of calming acid reflux

Alongside working on your energy field, it is helpful to look at what you eat. I have worked with the energy of a number of clients who suffer with the uncomfortable complaint of acid reflux and find great benefit from eating small meals, little and often. They may consume a light snack, perhaps an apple, between breakfast and lunch, and again between lunch and the evening meal. Sufferers should eat earlier in the evening and in smaller amounts (serving meals on a side plate helps you to become accustomed to smaller portions). Think about what foods you find hard to digest and that trigger acid, and reduce your intake of these or choose more gut-friendly alternatives. You may have to actively train your gut to reduce its acid production, so make wise food choices. Eating fruit can deliver a more positive acid for the gut. I have known people who have benefited from enjoying a cube of fresh (not canned) pineapple before retiring to bed, as this contains the enzyme group known as bromelain, which help to alleviate acid. A teaspoon of live yogurt (dairy or plant) eaten before bed can also help to calm acid. For the crystal configuration, use a tray or shoebox lid to support the coil formation of crystals, which is placed over the gut. Rose quartz is used for its energetic healing ability to deliver greater energetic peace, together with kyanite for energetically strengthening the body and bringing the alignment of the four lower bodies into greater harmony and flow. Program the crystals by asking:

> "I call upon the Light (or the earth energies), please charge these crystals with the highest positive energy to bring the digestive flow of (full name) into energetic peace, harmony, balance, and alignment. I thank the Light."

To begin energy work on the gut, I would recommend that anyone suffering from blockages or an imbalance in digestive flow contacts a soul recall therapist (alongside accessing medical help for their physical body) to gain some understanding of why they are afflicted

Fig. 28. The energy of calming acid reflux

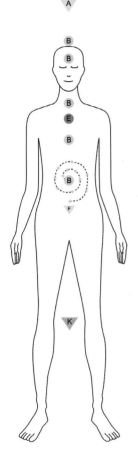

A =	ignitor crystal	12 inches (30 cm) above the crown chakra
B =	rose quartz	1 inch (2.5 cm) above the crown chakra
B =	rose quartz	third eye chakra
B =	rose quartz	throat chakra
E =	blue kyanite	thymus (halfway between the throat and heart chakras)
B =	rose quartz	heart chakra
B =	13 rose quartz	coil formation with a center rose quartz sited between the solar plexus and sacral chakras
F =	1 quartz crystal	single-terminated, beneath the last rose quartz in the coil, directed toward the exit crystal
K =	exit crystal	between the knees

Crystal energy healing time: 10 minutes
Aftercare: rest, drink water, and (if time allows) bathe or shower
Repeat session: twice a month
Notes: fasten the crystals in place on a shoebox lid / tray using microporous tape, then place the lid on the body, perhaps supported at the sides with cushions in order to keep the crystals level and in formation.

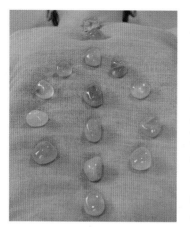

in this way. Wearing a programmed kyanite can be very helpful, as this crystal promotes strength, harmony, and balance in the physical body. In addition, having regular crystal healing for chakra balancing with the inclusion of rose quartz and amethyst at the site of the energy block can help to get stagnant energy moving from the energy field.

(Food intolerance or patterns of denial of food can be looked at to gain a greater understanding of the root cause through soul recall.)

The energy of irritable bowel syndrome (IBS)

When laying out crystal configurations on the body, it can be helpful to tape the crystals onto the contours of the skin in order to ensure their correct placement, but with layouts on the gut area, I find it easier to use a lightweight tray, a lap tray with a cushion attached, or indeed a box lid, with the crystal configuration already laid out and then simply placed gently on the stomach. A cushion positioned on either side of the body can help to secure the tray and make it feel more comfortable.

The crystal layout for an irritable bowel involves a coil of 12 small tumbled rose quartz crystals applied in a clockwise direction, spiraling out from a fluorite crystal placed over the abdomen, as shown. I put this part of the crystal configuration on a tray or lid, as mentioned, in order to prevent the crystals from rolling around when placed on the body. The remainder of the crystals in this configuration are positioned on or beyond the body, as shown. This crystal energy healing is suitable for use twice a month until the body feels more balanced. Crystals can be programmed by asking:

Fig. 29. The energy of irritable bowel syndrome (IBS)

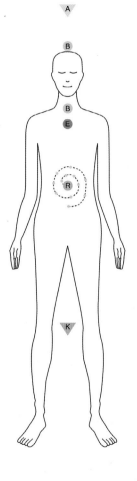

A =	ignitor crystal	12 inches (30 cm) above the crown chakra
B =	rose quartz	1 inch (2.5 cm) above the crown chakra
B =	rose quartz	throat chakra
E =	blue kyanite	thymus (halfway between the throat and heart chakras)
R =	fluorite crystal	between the solar plexus and sacral chakras
B =	12 rose quartz	in a coil formation, spiraling out from the fluorite (start of the coil)
K =	exit crystal	between the knees

Crystal energy healing time: 10 minutes
Aftercare: rest, drink water, and (if time allows) bathe or shower
Repeat session: twice a month
Notes: use a large shoebox lid or a tray to support the placement of crystals in the correct coil formation and direction.

"I call upon the Light (or the earth energies), please charge these crystals to bring energetic healing, peace, calm, and harmonious flow to the digestive system of (full name). I thank the Light."

The energy of constipation

What energy are you holding on to and simply cannot let go? Soul recall will bring some understanding of the root of the difficulty, and in conjunction with crystal healing, will help to release the energy blockages. The crystal layout for constipation is very similar to the layout for an irritable bowel, using the same programmed crystals in configuration. This energetic crystal layout can be used daily until balanced flow has resumed. Program the crystal by asking:

"I call upon the Light (or earth energies), please charge these crystals to bring greater energetic flow and release within the digestive system of (full name) so that (full name) may be of greater energetic peace, harmony, and alignment. I thank the Light."

Fig. 30. The energy of constipation

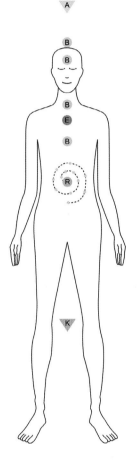

A =	ignitor crystal	12 inches (30 cm) above the crown chakra
B =	rose quartz	1 inch (2.5 cm) above the crown chakra
B =	rose quartz	third eye chakra
B =	rose quartz	throat chakra
E =	blue kyanite	thymus (halfway between the throat and heart chakras)
B =	rose quartz	heart chakra
R =	fluorite crystal	between the solar plexus and sacral chakra
B =	12 rose quartz	coil formation following the fluorite (start of the coil)
K =	exit crystal	between the knees

Crystal energy healing time: 10 minutes

Aftercare: rest, drink water, and (if time allows) bathe or shower

Repeat session: can be repeated daily until balanced flow returns

Notes: use a large box lid or a tray to support the placement of crystals in the correct coil formation and direction.

The energy of strengthening for GORD (gastroesophageal reflux dis-ease)

Always check this condition with your doctor. Many of my clients suffering from long bouts of acid reflux have experienced a common digestive complaint—a disorder of the lower esophageal sphincter, where the most typical symptoms are heartburn and acid reflux. Amethyst crystals are used in this crystal healing, together with kyanite, in a similar way to crystal healing for acid reflux. Amethyst builds and strengthens the energy, absorbing negative, stuck energy and igniting energetic flow to the area. To strengthen the energy of the sphincter, program the crystals by asking:

"I call upon the Light (or earth energies), please charge these crystals with the highest positive energy to bring the digestive flow of (full name) into greater strength of energetic peace, calm, and alignment. I thank the Light."

Fig. 31. The energy of strengthening for GORD (gastroesophageal reflux dis-ease)

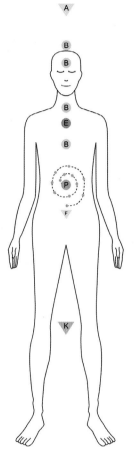

A =	ignitor crystal	12 inches (30 cm) above the crown chakra
B =	rose quartz	1 inch (2.5 cm) above the crown chakra
B =	rose quartz	third eye chakra
B =	rose quartz	throat chakra
E =	blue kyanite	thymus (halfway between the throat and heart chakras)
B =	rose quartz	heart chakra
P =	13 amethyst	coil formation with the center amethyst (start of the coil) sited between the solar plexus and sacral chakras
F =	1 quartz crystal	single-terminated (directed toward the exit crystal) beneath the last amethyst in the coil
K =	exit crystal	between the knees

Crystal energy healing time: 10 minutes
Aftercare: rest, drink water, and (if time allows) bathe or shower
Repeat session: twice a month
Notes: use a large shoebox lid or a tray to support the placement of crystals in the correct coil formation and direction.

The energy of happy gut health

To support a positive flow of energy, carry or wear a programmed fluorite, and always make sure you have your gut health checked out by a doctor. As we see in the news all too regularly, bowel cancer is difficult to detect, so be persistent if things do not improve or if you continue to feel unwell. Do not put off getting checked out. Ask for a stool test to check for a potential parasite. This may not always be high on the checklist, but it can be common if you travel to certain countries, so make sure your doctor knows about any overseas trips to ensure they test for this. If you are recovering from any kind of gut challenge, perhaps following a bout of illness, wearing or carrying a programmed fluorite can stimulate flow in the energy field. Use this beneficial crystal configuration once a week until the gut feels more balanced. Program the crystals by asking:

"I call upon the Light (or earth energies), please charge these crystals to positively energize the gut of (full name) so that their digestive system may be of greater peace, harmony, flow, and alignment. I thank the Light."

Fig. 32. The energy of happy gut health

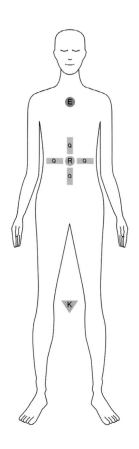

A =	ignitor crystal	12 inches (30 cm) above the crown chakra
E =	blue kyanite	thymus (halfway between the throat and heart chakras)
R =	fluorite	centered between the solar plexus and sacral chakras
Q =	4 selenite bars	north, south, east, west around the fluorite
K =	exit crystal	between the knees

Crystal energy healing time: 10 minutes
Aftercare: rest, drink water, and (if time allows) bathe or shower
Repeat session: once a week until the gut feels balanced and positive
Notes: selenite bars can be lightweight, and small selenite bars work just as effectively as larger ones from an energy perspective. Secure the crystals on the body with microporous tape.

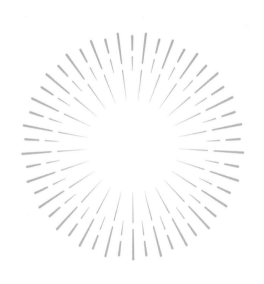

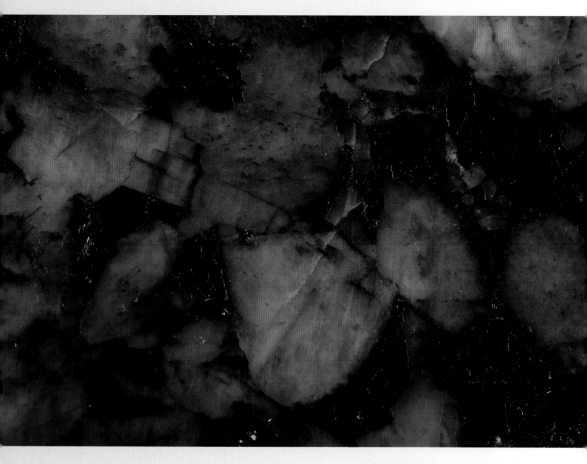

Chapter 7

The Immune
System and Sleep

The energy of allergies*

A sensitivity to life is the energetic root of an allergic reaction. In extreme circumstances such a reaction can be fatal. Greater understanding may be found through soul recall therapy, which can help to shift the blocked energy through acknowledgment. Crystal work can then begin to move the energy blocks even more. From an energetic perspective, the aim of this crystal healing is to align the heart to the head, along with the alignment of the four lower bodies in harmony to the soul path. Note the inclusion of green and blue kyanite in the crystal configuration. Together they have a multidimensional alchemy of energy: blue kyanite works on strengthening the alignment of the energy of the four lower bodies to the Light, and green kyanite works on empowering the alignment of the systems of the physical body (the digestive and vascular systems, and so on), aligning these to the energy of the chakra system for a more harmonious flow of energy. Together they have an empowered energy, like musical notes in a perfectly paired harmony, powering up the energy field in strengthened, aligned flow. The crystal layout shown here can be employed weekly until symptoms improve. You can program it by asking:

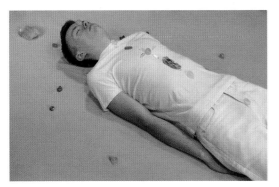

> "I call upon the Light (or earth energies) to transmute the pattern of negativity that manifests as an allergic reaction from (full name) so that greater positive flow of the four lower bodies in the energy of peace, harmony, and alignment may prevail. I thank the Light."

* For all health challenges please seek advice from a physical doctor to go hand in hand with the energy therapy you undertake.

Fig. 33. The energy of allergies

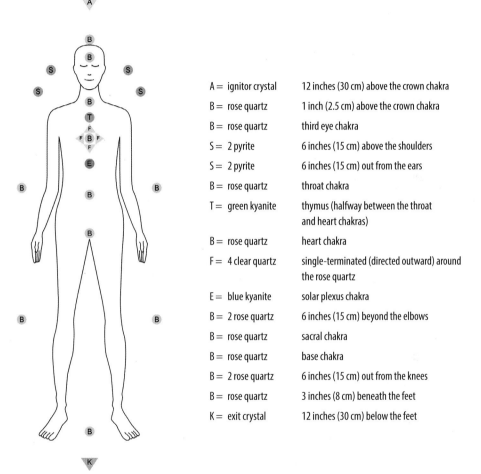

A = ignitor crystal   12 inches (30 cm) above the crown chakra

B = rose quartz   1 inch (2.5 cm) above the crown chakra

B = rose quartz   third eye chakra

S = 2 pyrite   6 inches (15 cm) above the shoulders

S = 2 pyrite   6 inches (15 cm) out from the ears

B = rose quartz   throat chakra

T = green kyanite   thymus (halfway between the throat and heart chakras)

B = rose quartz   heart chakra

F = 4 clear quartz   single-terminated (directed outward) around the rose quartz

E = blue kyanite   solar plexus chakra

B = 2 rose quartz   6 inches (15 cm) beyond the elbows

B = rose quartz   sacral chakra

B = rose quartz   base chakra

B = 2 rose quartz   6 inches (15 cm) out from the knees

B = rose quartz   3 inches (8 cm) beneath the feet

K = exit crystal   12 inches (30 cm) below the feet

Crystal energy healing time: 10 minutes

Aftercare: rest, drink water, and (if time allows) bathe or shower

Repeat session: twice a month

Notes: for layouts/grids such as this, which involve many crystals, take your time placing them on and around the body. Begin with the ignitor crystal, then the exit crystal, and then slowly and carefully place the remaining crystals as required from the head to the feet.

The energy of protecting and strengthening the immune system

The strength of our immune system is very important; it is how we tackle challenges such as illness, allergies, and infection in our body. To strengthen the energy of your immune system, begin by wearing or carrying programmed amethyst and labradorite crystals on alternate days. The amethyst cleanses and boosts the energy of the whole four lower bodies and the labradorite stimulates the immune system, energetically retuning, refining, and rebooting it (if required and appropriate to the life plan). Introduce a crystal energy healing configuration as shown, programmed by asking:

> *"I call upon the Light (or earth energies), please charge these crystals with the highest positive energy to bring harmony, balance, and alignment to the immune system of (full name). I thank the Light."*

A great many energy challenges surround us on our planet today. Wearing or carrying programmed amethyst and labradorite crystals on alternate days creates an energy veil or bubble, which helps to strengthen the energy field and can be programmed **for energetic protection** by asking:

> *"I call upon the Light, (or earth energies), please charge these crystals with the highest positive energy to protect and strengthen the energy field of (full name). I thank the Light."*

Fig. 34. The energy of protecting and strengthening the immune system

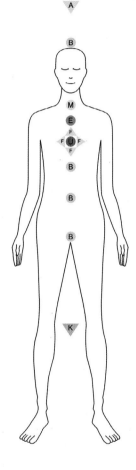

A = ignitor crystal   12 inches (30 cm) above the crown chakra

B = rose quartz   1 inch (2.5 cm) above the crown chakra

M = citrine   throat chakra

E = blue kyanite   thymus (halfway between the throat and heart chakras)

U = labradorite   heart chakra

F = 4 clear quartz   single-terminated (directed outward) around rthe ose quartz

B = rose quartz   solar plexus chakra

B = rose quartz   sacral chakra

B = rose quartz   base chakra

K = exit crystal   between the knees

Crystal energy healing time: 10 minutes
Aftercare: rest, drink water, and (if time allows) bathe or shower
Repeat session: weekly as required.

The energy of infection

The crystal layout/grid for purifying blood is a good place to start energy work. The diagram opposite shows the placement of crystals on and around the body in the case of a localized infection (such as of the chest or feet). The crystals will absorb negative energy from the energy field, igniting a positive charge and thereby supporting the active transmutation of energy that encourages a healing flow. Program crystals by asking:

> "I call upon the Light (or the earth energies), please charge these crystals with the highest positive energy to bring the healing energetic flow of transmutation, rejuvenation, and regeneration to (full name). I thank the Light."

Fig. 35. The energy of infection – chest

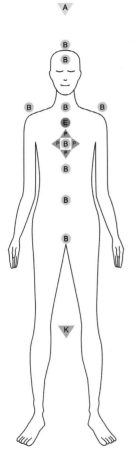

A =	ignitor crystal	12 inches (30 cm) above the crown chakra
B =	rose quartz	1 inch (2.5 cm) above the crown chakra
B =	rose quartz	third eye chakra
B =	rose quartz	throat chakra
B =	2 rose quartz	1 inch (2.5 cm) above each shoulder
E =	blue kyanite	thymus (halfway between the throat and heart chakras)
B =	rose quartz	heart chakra
P =	4 amethyst	single-terminated (directed outward) around the rose quartz (heart)
B =	rose quartz	solar plexus chakra
B =	rose quartz	sacral chakra
B =	rose quartz	base chakra
K =	exit crystal	between the knees

Crystal energy healing time: 10 minutes
Aftercare: rest, drink water, and (if time allows) bathe or shower
Repeat session: every two days as required, then twice a week. Continue this energy healing twice a month until the energy is clear and feels replenished.

Fig. 36. The energy of infection – foot

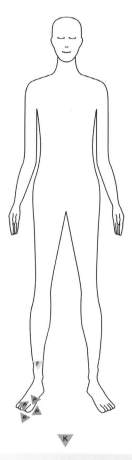

A =	ignitor crystal	12 inches (30 cm) above the crown chakra
F =	quartz crystal	single-terminated, directed toward the site of infection
P =	4 amethyst	single-terminated, around the site of infection
K =	exit crystal	12 inches (30 cm) below the feet

Crystal energy healing time: 10 minutes
Aftercare: rest, drink water, and (if time allows) bathe or shower
Repeat session: every other day as required, until the energy is clear and replenished
Notes: it is important to take note of the direction of the amethyst single-terminated points, as their placement directs the flow of energy. Positive energy is directed through the site of infection toward the absorber of negative energy, the exit crystal.

The energy of enhanced sleep

Our quality of sleep is so impacted today that it has spawned an entire industry. Trade shows that are open to the public sell and advise on anything and everything connected to our sleep, or our lack of it. Sleep is very important energetically. During sleep we rest the body and reconnect to the Light if we are functioning at our most positive. Energetic sleep has a timed rhythm to its process; if we are out of sync with this rhythm, our sleep is impacted. We "miss the sleepy train," as my Light friends tell me. When our sleep is negatively impacted, we do not get the quality of rest, reconnection, and Light rejuvenation that we are designed by the Light to achieve. This is not a huge problem if it occurs once or twice, but increasingly I encounter people who seem to have no quality sleep at all. This has a negative impact on one's whole energy health. I have firsthand experience of people who cannot sleep due to high levels of pain from injury or illness. In such cases holistic solutions can deliver some proper rest.

For a truly enhanced sleep we must follow a positive sleep pattern. When I talk to clients who are unable to sleep, I discover that many engage in very counterproductive activity prior to sleep and then wonder why it eludes them. Watching television until the early hours and viewing negative energy videos or movies (horror films, for example) are not positive or conducive to a good night's sleep. Alcohol used to aid sleep is not a positive solution, nor is medication, as ultimately your body gets used to these and you begin to require increasing amounts to achieve the desired result, which will be sleep of a kind, but not positive energy-enhanced sleep. Zoning out by scrolling on your phone or tablet or catching up with something on your laptop does not encourage positive energy-enhanced sleep.

A positive regime from an energetic perspective involves preparing your energy to sleep with, for example, some gentle yoga stretches an hour before bed, a warming oat milk drink, a warm bath with a drop of quality lavender oil, or reading something light and positive in content. Aim to be in bed in time to catch the sleepy train leaving at 10pm. Some of you may balk at attempting to be asleep by this hour. From an energetic perspective sleep establishes a flow: rest, reconnection, and rejuvenation. Positive energetic sleep finds you awake, aware, and ready to meet the day, bright and breezy, early the next morning because you have allowed your body to rest, your spirit to reconnect to the Light, and enough time for your energy field to rejuvenate. Your daily "bread" (or karma) envelops you during the dawn period and you meet the day's karma far more positively after a positive energetic sleep. You may not manage to introduce this kind of sleep into your routine seven nights a week, but aim to have at least three to four nights a week of quality sleep and you will feel the difference. Positive sleep requires practice if you have adopted negative sleep habits. It takes time and positive energy practice to undo what you have trained your body to do until now, which is to *not* sleep, so implement the new routines described to realign your energy patterns. It will be worth it. The saying "early to bed, early to rise, makes a man healthy, wealthy, and wise" is all too true.

Adding positive vibrational energy to make your bedroom a calm space, a sleep sanctuary, can also help. Plain white bedding in natural fibers carries a higher vibration, a purer vibration that adds to the positive, sleep-supporting energy. A rose quartz circuit (four rose quartz crystals programmed and placed in the four corners of the bedroom) will help envelop the space in the Light of peace. Keep the room aligned (tidy and clean). Positive vibrational energy flow likes clean, clear spaces and dislikes clutter, which catches energy and creates stagnation. Take care what you put under your bed. If you use it for storage, make sure it is neat, tidy, and free of anything negative that might affect your positive sleep vibrationally.

Programmed rose quartz crystals, either worn or carried, help the energy field by introducing a greater energy of the vibration of peace. A flat massage stone of rose quartz can be programmed in the same

Fig. 37. The energy of enhanced sleep

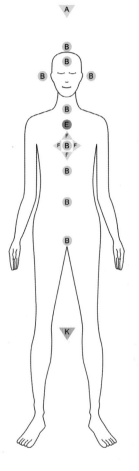

A =	ignitor crystal	12 inches (30 cm) above the crown chakra
B =	rose quartz	1 inch (2.5 cm) above the crown chakra
B =	rose quartz	third eye chakra
B =	rose quartz	3 inches (8 cm) beyond the ears
B =	rose quartz	throat chakra
E =	blue kyanite	thymus (halfway between the throat and heart chakras)
B =	rose quartz	heart chakra
F =	4 clear quartz	single-terminated (directed outward) around the rose quartz (heart)
B =	rose quartz	solar plexus chakra
B =	rose quartz	sacral chakra
B =	rose quartz	base chakra
K =	exit crystal	between the knees

Crystal energy healing time: 10 minutes

Aftercare: rest, drink water, and (if time allows) bathe or shower

Repeat session: weekly for a month, then repeat as required

Notes: this crystal energy healing facilitates the energy of peace and alignment in your energy field. With regular crystal energy healing, the greater the flow of your energy, the greater the flow of your potential energy harmony and balance, therefore the greater the flow to the ability and opportunity to enjoy a positive quality of sleep.

way and placed under your pillow at night to encourage positive, restful, and peaceful sleep. A weekly crystal energy healing configuration can be introduced as shown, with the crystals programmed by asking:

"I call upon the Light (or the earth energies), please charge these crystals with the highest positive energy to promote peaceful, restful, Light-reconnecting and Light-rejuvenating sleep for (full name). I thank the Light."

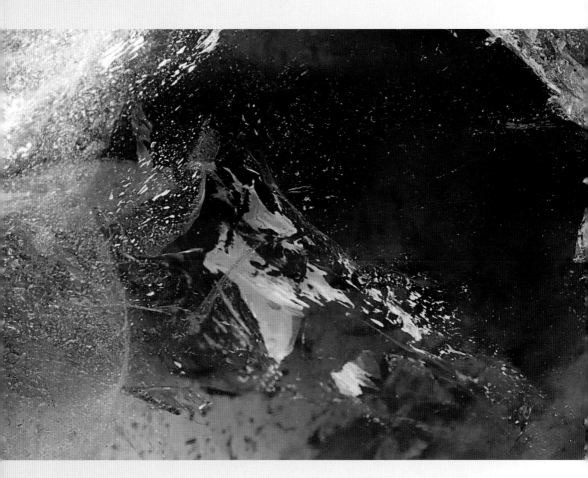

Chapter 8

The Skin and Hair

The energy of enhanced skin

For many, the holy grail of beauty is flawless and fabulous skin, but it is a universal truth that beauty comes from within. True beauty is the beauty of the energy you reflect in its totality. You may possess so-called conventional beauty according to contemporary norms, which change over time, of course, but if you are manifesting an energy of negativity (perhaps you are self-focused at the expense of some or many of those around you), negative energy patterns will

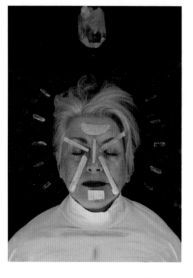

begin to manifest over your physicality. Add to this the toxic nature of our surroundings, the food we ingest, the drinks we imbibe, the chemicals we use and to which we are exposed, and we are rapidly eroding the gifts we have been dealt in the beauty stakes. Energy cleansing is positive only if you also work at supporting it by keeping your physical body well cleansed: drink water, exercise, move your energy in your preferred way, and make sure you get plenty of fresh air. Uplift your energy by being with people and in places that raise your spirits. Get regular crystal chakra balancing. All of these actions enhance the whole energy field and help you to manifest a greater beauty in the total energy you reflect to the world.

Selenite and rose quartz partner in this crystal configuration. Choose very lightweight, thin bars of selenite, and rest these on the face or gently secure them in position with microporous tape. Program the crystals by asking:

"I call upon the Light (or earth energies), please charge these crystals with the highest positive vibration of energetic peace and healing to replenish and nourish the skin of (full name). I thank the Light."

Fig. 38. The energy of enhanced skin

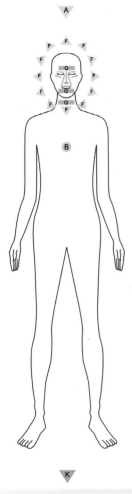

A = ignitor crystal   12 inches (30 cm) above the crown chakra

Q = selenite bars   arranged on the face

F = 12 clear quartz   single-terminated (directed outward), 3 inches (8 cm) beyond the head

B = rose quartz   heart chakra

K = exit crystal   12 inches (30 cm) below the feet

Crystal energy healing time: 10 minutes
Aftercare: rest, drink water, and (if time allows) bathe or shower
Repeat session: monthly
Notes: selenite bars can be secured gently and carefully on the face, or if the skin is sensitive, arranged on a clean, lightweight natural fiber cloth, which is then placed over the face, again secured if necessary with microporous tape.

The energy of the skin on the face

Rose quartz facilitates the energy of greater peace. The skin is our protective organ, so if we have a skin complaint, metaphysical understanding tells us that we are carrying the energy of some kind of vulnerability, that there is a conflict of energy within our protective organ, the skin. Start by wearing or carrying rose quartz programmed to envelop the person concerned with the highest Light of peace to their energy field. For adults, wearing rose quartz over the heart chakra is best. For children, place the programmed crystal in the room in which they spend most time, or put the crystal in a pouch and secure it in the pocket of a garment they like to wear. This can be very beneficial to their energy well-being. Be aware that small crystals and small children do not go together well. If the child is under twelve, I would suggest programming a larger piece, for example a rose quartz of sufficient size that it cannot be put in the mouth or up the nose, as we know some children like to do. Place the crystal well out of reach on a shelf in a bedroom or living space.

The diagram explains the crystal layout for energy healing for the head and face, but it could be set up in a similar fashion for other areas of the body that are experiencing a localized outbreak, such as an elbow or knee. Program the crystal layout for **energy healing the head/face** by asking:

"I call upon the Light (or the earth energies), please charge these crystals with the highest positive energy to align, heal, and regenerate the skin of (full name). I thank the Light."

There is an alternative crystal configuration in which the crystals do not touch the skin. I have worked with people whose skin is so sore and inflamed (often from an energy related to a burn) that it would be too painful to have crystals resting directly on their skin. In this instance, very clean, natural fiber cloths (preferably cotton) can be placed over the area and small, lightweight crystals applied gently on top.

Fig. 39. The energy of the skin on the face

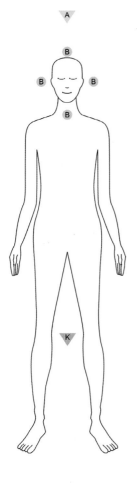

A = ignitor crystal   12 inches (30 cm) above the crown chakra

B = rose quartz   1 inch (2.5 cm) above the crown chakra

B = rose quartz   2 inches (5 cm) beyond each ear

B = rose quartz   throat chakra

K = exit crystal   between the knees

Crystal energy healing time: 10 minutes
Aftercare: rest, drink water, and (if time allows) bathe or shower
Repeat session: weekly.

The energy of the skin on the hands

Program the crystal layout for **energy healing the hands** by asking:

> "I call upon the Light (or earth energies), please charge these crystals with the highest positive energy to align, heal, and regenerate the skin of (full name). I thank the Light."

Fig. 40. The energy of the skin on the hands

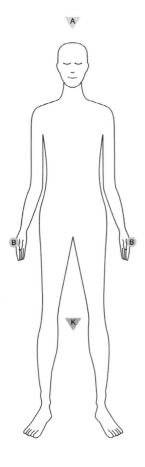

A = ignitor crystal   8 inches (20 cm) above the crown chakra

B = rose quartz   as required for the affected area,
or 1 crystal centered on the affected area

K = exit crystal   between the knees

Crystal energy healing time: 10 minutes
Aftercare: rest, drink water, and (if time allows) bathe or shower
Repeat session: weekly
Notes: take care if the hands are sore or if the skin is broken. It can help to place a clean, natural fiber cloth (such as cotton) over the affected area and to arrange lightweight crystals on the cloth.

The energy of face acne

Blemishes on the skin are painful in many ways. They can be acutely uncomfortable and tend to occur most at a time when a young person is beginning to "face" the world. The energy revealed is often anger, which manifests through the skin. You literally face the world with your anger. Rose quartz, the ultimate bringer of the energy of peace, is the crystal that resonates best in this situation. The first diagram illustrates how to energy charge the skin of the face and the second explains how to energy charge damaged skin on the back. I have had clients with both types of skin challenge, and they can be extremely painful. Program the crystals by asking:

"I call upon the Light (or earth energies), please charge these crystals with the highest positive energy of peace, harmony, and balance to bring alignment and energetic healing flow to (full name). I thank the Light."

Fig. 41. The energy of face acne

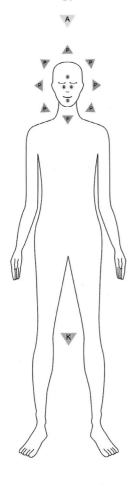

A = ignitor crystal   12 inches (30 cm) above the crown chakra

B = 4 rose quartz   on the face

P = 8 amethyst   single-terminated (directed outward)
3 inches (8 cm) beyond the head

K = exit crystal   between the knees

Crystal energy healing time: 10 minutes
Aftercare: rest, drink water, and (if time allows) bathe or shower
Repeat session: weekly
Notes: small pieces of rose quartz can be carefully secured to the contours of the face using microporous tape.

The energy of back acne

"I call upon the Light (or the earth energies), please charge these crystals with the highest positive energy of peace, harmony, and balance to bring alignment and energetic healing flow to (full name). I thank the Light."

Fig. 42. The energy of back acne

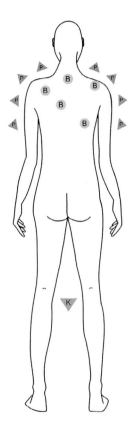

A = ignitor crystal   12 inches (30 cm) above the crown chakra

B = rose quartz   as many as required for the affected area

P = 8 amethyst   single-terminated (directed outward),
3 inches (8 cm) beyond the body

K = exit crystal   between the knees

Crystal energy healing time: 10 minutes
Aftercare: rest, drink water, and (if time allows) bathe or shower
Repeat session: weekly
Notes: rose quartz may be gently placed on the affected areas of the skin (as shown).

The energy of scars

When scars have healed (exposing no broken skin), an application of vitamin E oil can be of help alongside regular crystal energy healing where a combination of rose quartz and selenite crystals are used to promote the energy of skin healing and regeneration. Program the crystals by asking:

> "I call upon the Light (or the earth energies), please charge these crystals with the highest positive energy to ignite the energetic healing in the skin of (full name). I thank the Light."

Fig. 43. The energy of scars

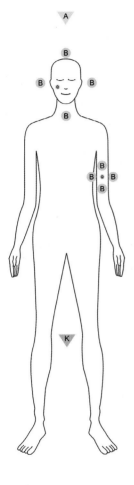

A =	ignitor crystal	12 inches (30 cm) above the crown chakra
B =	rose quartz	1 inch (2.5 cm) above the crown chakra
Q =	selenite bar	for example, over a facial scar
B =	rose quartz	2 inches (5 cm) beyond each ear
B =	rose quartz	throat chakra
Q =	selenite bar	for example, over a scar on the arm
B =	4 rose quartz	2–3 inches (5–8 cm) beyond the scar
K =	exit crystal	between the knees

Crystal energy healing time: 10 minutes
Aftercare: rest, drink water, and (if time allows) bathe or shower
Repeat session: weekly
Notes: crystals on the face or body can be carefully secured in position with microporous tape.

The energy of replenishing and strengthening thinning or weak hair

In the early stages of hair loss, it is important to distinguish it from alopecia. For weakened hair roots, there is a greater possibility of stimulating growth energetically. Alopecia is a much more extreme hair loss condition and, together with consulting your doctor, it requires greater energetic work to achieve an understanding and integration of the energetic causes. Try to find a direct connection to a holistic soul recall therapist in order to gain a personal under-standing of what is happening energetically. Thinning, weakened hair benefits from energetic stimulation to displace the stagnant energy from the energy field. Program the crystals by asking:

"I call upon the Light (or earth energies), please charge these crys-tals with the highest positive energy that they may bring healing energy to the hair follicles and ignite the healing growth and strength of hair for (full name) at this time. I thank the Light."

Fig. 44. The energy of replenishing and strengthening thinning or weak hair

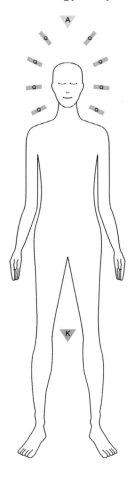

A = ignitor crystal   12 inches (30 cm) above the crown chakra

Q = 8 selenite bars   4 inches (10 cm) beyond the head

K = exit crystal   between the knees

Crystal energy healing time: 10 minutes
Aftercare: rest, drink water, and (if time allows) bathe or shower
Repeat session: weekly.

Holistic tips

Incorporate scalp massage into this weekly crystal treatment, perhaps with the help of friends and family. Every three days massage a mixture of good quality olive oil (a tablespoon) and three drops of vitamin E oil into your scalp to stimulate blood flow to the hair follicles. After the massage wear a head-scarf or towel turban overnight. This warms the oil and encourages absorption into the hair follicles and skin, giving the oil extra time to do its work. Wash off the oil residue the next morning. Take care to use natural shampoos and con-ditioners, and try not to overwork or the hair or style it too much.

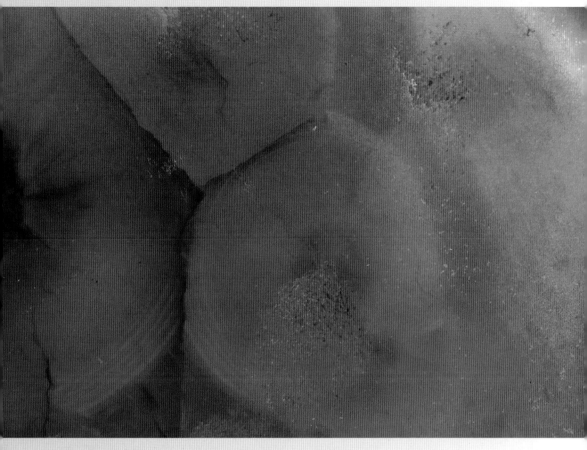

Chapter 9

The Head

The energy of tinnitus

From an energetic perspective, tinnitus manifests in the inner ear when the individual is unwilling to return to balance in life. Greater understanding can come through soul recall therapy, followed by working with crystals to absorb the negative energy that has accumulated around the ear. Crystals can be programmed by asking:

> *"I call upon the Light (or earth energies), please charge these crystals to bring peace, flow, balance, harmony, and alignment to the energy of (full name's) ears and hearing. I thank the Light."*

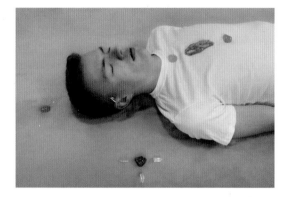

Fig. 45. The energy of tinnitus

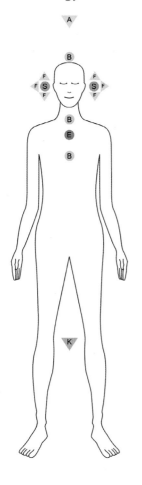

A =	ignitor crystal	12 inches (30 cm) above the crown chakra
B =	rose quartz	1 inch/2.5 cm above the crown chakra
S =	pyrite	3 inches (8 cm) beyond the ears
F =	6 clear quartz	single-terminated (directed outward) around the pyrite
B =	rose quartz	throat chakra
E =	blue kyanite	thymus (halfway between the throat and heart chakras)
B =	rose quartz	heart chakra
K =	exit crystal	between the knees

Crystal energy healing time: 10 minutes
Aftercare: rest, drink water, and (if time allows) bathe or shower
Repeat session: weekly as required.

The energy of headaches (sinus)

Rose quartz is the ultimate bringer of the energy of peace, as already mentioned. Program the crystal layout/grid for **energy healing a headache** by asking:

> *"I call upon the Light (or earth energies), please charge these crystals with the highest positive energy of peace for the energy transmutation and energy healing of (full name) at this time. I thank the Light."*

Energy healing for a headache does not require the use of an ignitor crystal, since this would in fact increase the volume of energy and could potentially add to the intensity of the headache. Instead, draw the negative energy from the head down toward the exit crystal, where it can be absorbed and transmuted. Without the ignitor crystal, this is a gentler healing experience that also disperses the energy connected to the headache.

Note: Sinus pain is unpleasant. The spaces located within the bones of the skull serve to lighten the skull. The lining of these spaces secretes mucus, which should flow out under normal circumstances, but when mucus resists and fails to drain it can be very painful. The clue, as ever, to the metaphysical cause of this pain is establishing its location. Is it the teeth, nose, or eyes? If it is due to an energy retention or blockage, which decisions are you not making (teeth)? What are you not observing that is right in front of you (nose)? What are you not seeing? Are you failing to release negative patterns of past experiences (past life)? Mucus is a release of toxins through the body, so something in the energy of your life has "flushed up" for you to clear. If the pain is confined to the bridge of the nose, it points to the energy of family issues (the bridge between you and your family members). What needs to be bridged in harmony and energetic healing? Sinus pain that manifests in the cheek suggests a challenge to the energy of how you view the world. How do you face it, and with what energy? (See page 132 for more ways to help with sinus pain.)

Fig. 46. The energy of headaches (sinus)

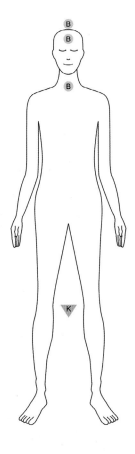

B = rose quartz   1 inch (2.5 cm) above the crown chakra

B = rose quartz   third eye chakra

B = rose quartz   throat chakra

K = exit crystal   between the knees

Crystal energy healing time: 10 minutes
Aftercare: rest, drink water, and (if time allows) bathe or shower
Repeat session: weekly
Notes: crystals on the face or body can be carefully secured in position with microporous tape.
No ignitor crystal is required as outlined.

The energy of clarity of vision

From an energy point of view, when light is unable to pass through the lens of the eye, it indicates the energy of a desire to block out the Light, to not witness or acknowledge the truth in some way, and a reluctance to witness the life ahead. You may see some truths but not those that you do not wish to see, so you must look at those aspects of your life that you are otherwise unwilling to examine.

Glaucoma involves a build-up of pressure in the eye. The receptors at the back of the eye interpret what you see, so from an energetic perspective, your eye and your nerves are speaking to you. Your inner sense has shut down and you have closed the energy of your heart.

A combination of selenite (for the energy of cellular regeneration) set within a single-terminated clear quartz crystal grid of energy can be programmed by asking:

> *"I call upon the Light (or the earth energies), please charge these crystals to revitalize the energy of the eyes to greater clarity of energetic positivity for (full name). I thank the Light."*

Fig. 47. The energy of clarity of vision

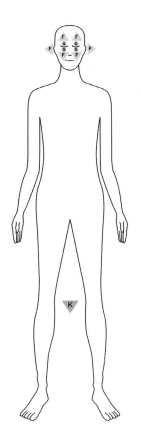

A = ignitor crystal   12 inches (30 cm) above the crown chakra

Q = 4 selenite bars   above and below each eye

F = 6 clear quartz   single-terminated (directed outward)
                                    above the eyebrows (x 2)
                                    below the eyes on the cheeks (x 2)
                                    1 inch (2.5 cm) beyond the head, in line
                                    with eyes (x 2)

K = exit crystal   between the knees

Crystal energy healing time: 10 minutes
Aftercare: rest, drink water, and (if time allows) bathe or shower
Repeat session: weekly
Notes: crystals placed on the face or body can be carefully secured in position with microporous tape.

The energy of blocked tear ducts (dry eyes)

Emerald crystal resonates to the blockage of energy in the eyes. If you have difficulty obtaining a small piece of rough emerald, use a small, lightweight rose quartz, or a flat but lightweight rose quartz massage stone instead. Avoid putting anything too heavy or uncomfortable directly onto the eye. A clean crystal can be placed directly on the skin, but for most clients, family members, or friends I recommend using a clean, lightweight fine cotton cloth that can be placed over the affected eye first, with the crystal placed on top of the cloth. It can be secured in position with microporous tape if necessary. Crystals can be programmed by asking:

> "I call upon the Light (or the earth energies), please charge these crystals to bring peace, flow, harmony, and alignment to the energy of (full name's) eye/s. I thank the Light."

Fig. 48. The energy of blocked tear ducts (dry eyes)

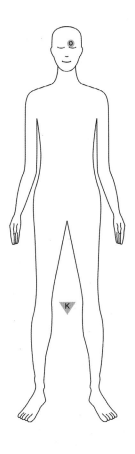

A = ignitor crystal   12 inches (30 cm) above the crown chakra

O = emerald   over the eye

OR

B = rose quartz   over the eye (crystal taped onto a clean cloth)

K = exit crystal   between the knees

Crystal energy healing time: 10 minutes
Aftercare: rest, drink water, and (if time allows) bathe or shower
Repeat session: weekly
Notes: crystals placed on the face or body can be carefully secured in position with microporous tape.

The energy of hearing

For some of us, our hearing is impaired during our lives for a soul purpose; some of us incur energy blocks when we stop listening to, and indeed really hearing, the people around us. Others collect blocks of energy in this area as we age. For those instances where change to the flow of energy can be implemented, program this crystal layout/grid by asking:

> "I call upon the Light (or the earth energies), please charge these crystals to bring peace, flow, harmony, and alignment to the energy of (full name's) ears and hearing. I thank the Light."

Fig. 49. The energy of hearing

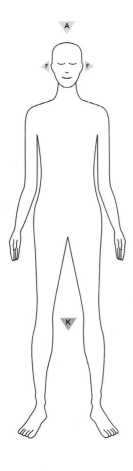

A = ignitor crystal   4 inches (10 cm) above the crown chakra

F = 2 clear quartz   single-terminated (directed outward)
2 inches (5 cm) beyond the ears

K = exit crystal   between the knees

Crystal energy healing time: 10 minutes
Aftercare: rest, drink water, and (if time allows) bathe or shower
Repeat session: weekly as required.

The energy of the teeth and gums

Of course, mouth and breath health, along with halitosis can be helped by good oral hygiene together with a balanced gut. Poor oral health can also manifest energetically from "bad-mouthing" in a literal sense, from talking negatively about people, things, and events. Crystals can help with mouth health energetically. Program the crystals by asking:

> "I call upon the Light (or the earth energies), please charge these crystals with the highest positive energy to cleanse, align, and balance the energy of (full name's) mouth at this time. I thank the Light."

Fig. 50. The energy of the teeth and gums

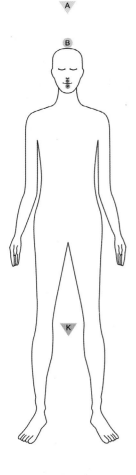

A =	ignitor crystal	12 inches (30 cm) above the crown chakra
B =	rose quartz	1 inch (2.5 cm) above the the crown chakra
B =	rose quartz	double-terminated above the top lip
P =	amethyst	double-terminated below the lower lip
K =	exit crystal	between the knees

Crystal energy healing time: 10 minutes
Aftercare: rest, drink water, and (if time allows) bathe or shower
Repeat session: as required
Notes: choose a small, flat tumbled piece of rose quartz that can be easily secured to the area of discomfort with microporous tape.

The energy of the teeth (mouth pain)

For oral health, dental pain or discomfort, dental surgery, and care after dental treatment, program crystals by asking:

"I call upon the Light (or earth energies), please charge these crystals to envelop the highest positive energy for peace and greater energetic healing to (full name) at this time. I thank the Light."

Fig. 51. The energy of the teeth (mouth pain)

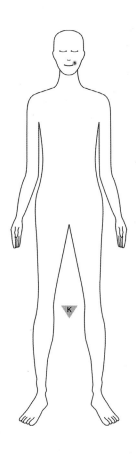

A = ignitor crystal   12 inches (30 cm) above the crown chakra
B = rose quartz   over the site of discomfort
K = exit crystal   between the knees

Crystal energy healing time: 10 minutes
Aftercare: rest, drink water, and (if time allows) bathe or shower
Repeat session: weekly as required
Notes: if double-terminated crystals are not available, use small tumbled pieces of rose quartz and amethyst instead.

The energy of the gums

Program crystals by asking:

"I call upon the Light (or the earth energies), please charge these crystals with the highest positive energy to bring energy healing, alignment, and balance to regenerate the gum health of (full name). I thank the Light."

Holistic tips

I recommend adding a drop of good quality tea tree oil (always choose a quality option) to a cup or small tumbler of water as a final rinse (do not swallow) after brushing your teeth. This is beneficial for oral health, as tea tree is a natural antiseptic with antifungal and antibacterial properties but does not harm your good bacteria.

The same solution of tea tree oil and water can help to energy cleanse the nose. Use the tip of a soft, clean cotton handkerchief (or the clean tip of your little finger, providing the nail is short) to dip into the solution and carefully wash the inner nasal cavity (do not push, scratch, or prod). One of my clients with damage to the nose regained his sense of smell by following this nasal cleansing method, coupled with crystal energy work.

The same solution is also effective when used as a daily or nightly gargle. Many germs take hold in the throat and regular gargling with a tea tree oil solution can help to promote gum, mouth, and throat health.

Fig. 52. The energy of the gums

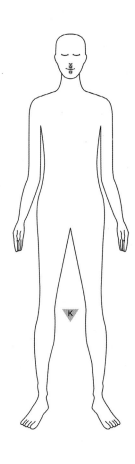

A =	ignitor crystal	12 inches (30 cm) above the crown chakra
Q =	2 selenite bars	above the top lip and below the lower lip
K =	exit crystal	between the knees

Crystal energy healing time: 10 minutes
Aftercare: rest, drink water, and (if time allows) bathe or shower
Repeat session: every 3 days or as required
Notes: crystals placed on the face or body can be carefully secured in position with microporous tape.

The energy of the nose (breathing freely and with flow)

If you are looking for evidence of just how closely connected your body is via its network of meridians, a blocked nose offers the perfect example. The next time you have a blocked nose, try pressing your pubic bone gently and hey presto! You will be able to breathe freely and with flow, but only for as long as you maintain light pressure on this point on the meridian circuit. This is a powerful demonstration of energetic change, of how we can free our energy as long as we know how to do so and have, of course, acknowledged that we actually *are* energy beings.

Ametrine crystal (a natural combination of amethyst and citrine) is an ideal energetic partner for moving blocked energy around the nose and sinuses through its ability to cleanse and absorb negative energy while flushing the area with positive energy and shifting energy from stagnation into flow.

Program crystals to promote breathing freely and with flow through the nose by saying:

> *"I call upon the Light (or earth energies), please charge these crystals to bring energetic healing flow to the nose and sinuses of (full name). I thank the Light."*

Fig. 53. The energy of the nose (breathing freely and with flow)

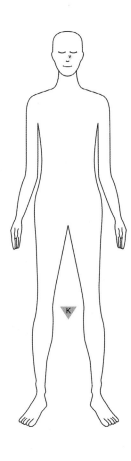

A = ignitor crystal   12 inches (30 cm) above the crown chakra

V = ametrine   on the site of discomfort

K = exit crystal   between the knees

Crystal energy healing time: 10 minutes
Aftercare: rest, drink water, and (if time allows) bathe or shower
Repeat session: daily until the discomfort subsides
Notes: it is helpful to sit or lie down and gently massage the sinuses/nose with the programmed ametrine to bring energetic relief to the site of the energy block.

The energy of the nose (sense of smell)

Selenite supports the energy of cellular regeneration and rose quartz creates an energy healing framework. Program the crystals by asking:

"I call upon the Light (or earth energies), please charge these crystals to bring the energy of healing regeneration and flow, enhancing the energy of sense of smell to the nose of (full name). I thank the Light."

Fig. 54. The energy of the nose (sense of smell)

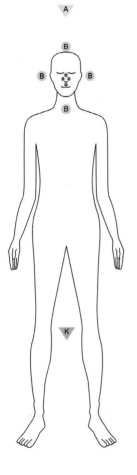

A =	ignitor crystal	12 inches (30 cm) above the crown chakra
B =	rose quartz	1 inch (2.5 cm) above the crown chakra
B =	2 rose quartz	1 inch (2.5 cm) beyond the ears
B =	2 rose quartz	either side of the nostrils
B =	rose quartz	throat chakra
Q =	selenite bar	bridge of the nose
Q =	selenite bar	above the top lip
K =	exit crystal	between the knees

Crystal energy healing time: 10 minutes
Aftercare: rest, drink water, and (if time allows) bathe or shower
Repeat session: weekly
Notes: crystals placed on the face or body can be carefully secured in position with microporous tape.

The energy of the jaw (alignment)

I worked with a client whose jaw clicked very loudly when he ate. Through energy work he realized that this was rooted in feelings of irritation, stress, and anger. Alongside holistic work on his emotions, to help energetically realign the jaw we used rose quartz in a crystal circuit, programmed by asking:

> "I call upon the Light (or earth energies), please charge these crystals so that they may be imbued with the highest positive energy to energetically align the jaw and face of (full name). I thank the Light."

Fig. 55. The energy of the jaw (alignment)

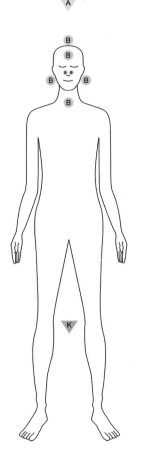

A =	ignitor crystal	12 inches (30 cm) above the crown chakra
B =	rose quartz	1 inch (2.5 cm) above the crown chakra
B =	rose quartz	third eye chakra
B =	2 rose quartz	1 inch (2.5 cm) beyond the head, just below the ears
B =	2 rose quartz	either side of the nostrils
B =	rose quartz	throat chakra
K =	exit crystal	between the knees

Crystal energy healing time: 10 minutes
Aftercare: rest, drink water, and (if time allows) bathe or shower
Repeat session: once a week until energy block alleviates, then twice a month
Notes: crystals placed on the face or body can be carefully secured in position with microporous tape.

The energy of the throat (alignment)

A blocked throat chakra is very common. So many of us "swallow" the things we really want to express and in doing so create a great energy "cap" that blocks the throat chakra. Eventually, this energy block manifests as physical symptoms such as a "frog in the throat," hoarseness, and so on. Throat chakra "toning" can help to release the block in conjunction with crystals. Toning the vibration of the OM mantra complements this energetic clearing. (Your voice will change in note and clarity as you continue to practice.) Program crystals by asking:

> *"I call upon the Light (or earth energies), please charge these crystals so that they may clear and open the energy of (full name's) throat chakra. I thank the Light."*

Fig. 56. The energy of the throat (alignment)

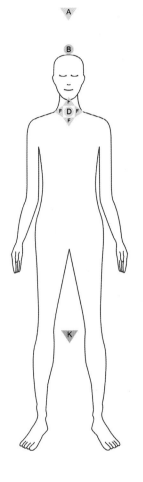

A = ignitor crystal   12 inches (30 cm) above the crown chakra

B = rose quartz   1 inch (2.5 cm) above the crown chakra

D = turquoise   throat chakra

F = clear quartz   single-terminated (directed outward) around the throat

K = exit crystal   between the knees

Crystal energy healing time: 10 minutes

Aftercare: rest, drink water, and (if time allows) bathe or shower

Repeat session: once a week until the energy block alleviates, then once a month

Notes: chanting the vibration of the OM can complement this energetic healing to clear blocks to the throat chakra. This crystal energy healing helps with having a "frog in the throat," hoarseness, weak energy of voice, and so on, caused by blocked energy.

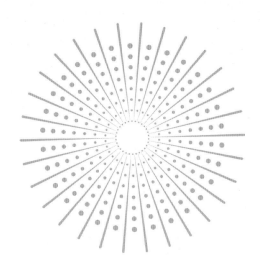

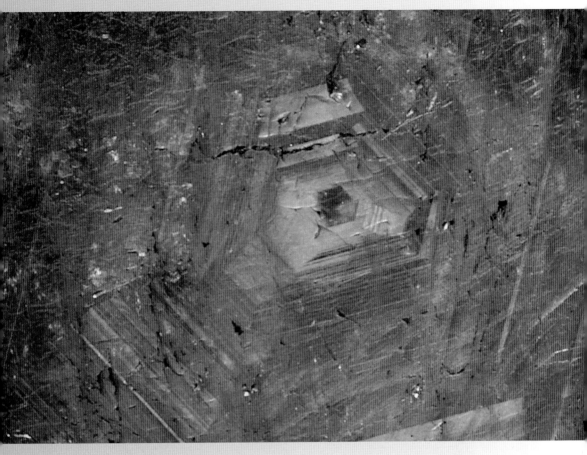

Chapter 10

Crystal Healing and the Energy of Dis-ease

The energy of Covid and long Covid

A dear friend of mine is a gifted energy intuitive and "sees" the human energy field by tuning in to "read" what is happening and what can be done energetically to restore optimum health. While discussing this book we began talking about Covid. My friend described how the energy of an individual yet to have Covid, who showed no

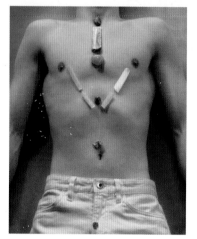

signs of it, and in whom the virus had not appeared in any way within the physical body but was energetically succumbing to Covid, was vividly apparent in the energy field around the head with a very obvious energy pattern of cylindrical, spiked clusters. These were the cylindrical, spiked clusters with which we all became so familiar in the news during the height of the pandemic. My friend informed me that these can be visible in the energy field well before the individual contracts Covid in the physical body. This example is a powerful indication of just how much there is to learn about the activity in our own human energy fields.

Crystals can create an energetic vibration, an alchemy of energy, to transmute negative energy within and without the body and throughout the energy field, in a way that can help Covid or long Covid sufferers (according to their life plan). The crystals required are labradorite, amethyst, citrine, rose quartz, and selenite (rose quartz works if selenite is not available).

For this alchemy of energy, a three-day cycle can be followed: on day one wear or carry programmed rose quartz, on day two wear or carry programmed amethyst, and on day three wear or carry programmed labradorite. Then repeat the three-day cycle until you no longer need to do so. The selenite bars can be programmed and placed on the lungs to regenerate the energy field where there is difficulty breathing or an issue of being short of or out of breath. Citrine can be programmed and placed in the home, charged to

Fig. 57. The energy of Covid and long Covid

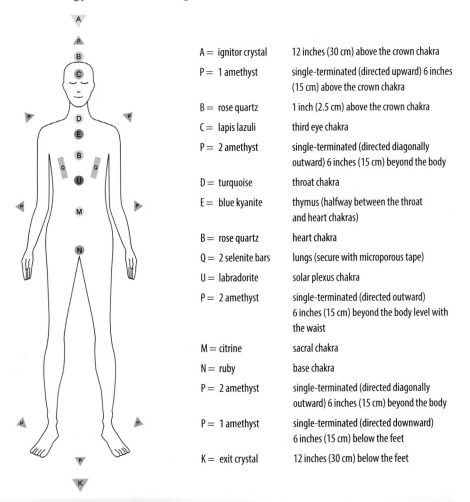

A = ignitor crystal — 12 inches (30 cm) above the crown chakra

P = 1 amethyst — single-terminated (directed upward) 6 inches (15 cm) above the crown chakra

B = rose quartz — 1 inch (2.5 cm) above the crown chakra

C = lapis lazuli — third eye chakra

P = 2 amethyst — single-terminated (directed diagonally outward) 6 inches (15 cm) beyond the body

D = turquoise — throat chakra

E = blue kyanite — thymus (halfway between the throat and heart chakras)

B = rose quartz — heart chakra

Q = 2 selenite bars — lungs (secure with microporous tape)

U = labradorite — solar plexus chakra

P = 2 amethyst — single-terminated (directed outward) 6 inches (15 cm) beyond the body level with the waist

M = citrine — sacral chakra

N = ruby — base chakra

P = 2 amethyst — single-terminated (directed diagonally outward) 6 inches (15 cm) beyond the body

P = 1 amethyst — single-terminated (directed downward) 6 inches (15 cm) below the feet

K = exit crystal — 12 inches (30 cm) below the feet

Crystal energy healing time: 10 minutes

Aftercare: rest, drink water, and (if time allows) bathe or shower

Repeat session: weekly as required

Notes: when laying out base chakra crystals on the body, it is helpful for purposes of placement, removal, and the preservation of dignity, to first place a thick towel on the relevant part of the body.

absorb and bring into positivity the energy around it. This means that the sufferer moves within, through, and around clear and regenerated energy in the home. A weekly crystal configuration of energy healing can follow, using a layout such as the one shown here, programmed by asking:

> "I call upon the Light (or earth energies), please charge these crystals with the highest positive energy to bring the Light of energetic transmutation and energetic healing to (full name). I thank the Light."

The energy of heart dis-ease

Begin by wearing or carrying a programmed rose quartz for a day and then alternate it with a programmed amethyst the next day. Continue alternating the two crystals for at least a month. They will work together in alchemical harmony to cleanse the energy field and the heart chakra, in combination with strengthening the latter and promoting more positive flow in the energy field where there is stagnant energy. You can then move on to crystal configuration layouts such as the one shown here. Program the crystals by asking:

> "I call upon the Light (or earth energies), please charge these crystals with the highest positive energy to promote energetic heart chakra healing, peace, harmony, alignment, and flow for (full name). I thank the Light."

Fig. 58. The energy of heart dis-ease

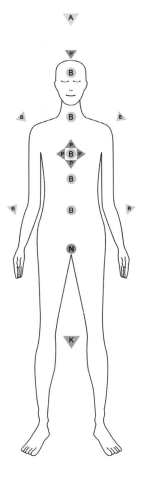

A =	ignitor crystal	12 inches (30 cm) above the crown chakra
P =	1 amethyst	single-terminated (directed downward) 1 inch (2.5 cm) above the crown chakra
B =	rose quartz	third eye chakra
B =	rose quartz	throat chakra
B =	4 rose quartz	single-terminated, 3 inches (8 cm) beyond the body, directed toward the heart chakra
B =	rose quartz	heart chakra
P =	4 amethyst	single-terminated (directed outward) around the rose quartz on the heart chakra
B =	rose quartz	solar plexus chakra
B =	rose quartz	sacral chakra
N =	ruby	base chakra
K =	exit crystal	between the knees

Crystal energy healing time: 10 minutes
Aftercare: rest, drink water, and (if time allows) bathe or shower
Repeat session: weekly as required
Notes: when laying out base chakra crystals on the body, it is helpful for purposes of placement, removal, and the preservation of dignity, to first place a thick towel on the relevant part of the body.

The energy of obsessive compulsory disorder (OCD)

Repetitive thoughts, compulsions, rituals, repeated checking, or checking a particular number of times result from the creation of a negative cycle of energy in which there is a fear of breaking out of the cycle. There is a desire not to change, which then imprisons the individual. This condition, known as OCD, is said to be up to twice as common in women as it is in men.

An obsession with cleanliness comes from a deep memory, an energetic "stain" from a past life that the person wishes to clear away. Connecting to the past memory through soul recall facilitates an understanding of why an individual is experiencing OCD at this time in their life, and this can be followed by a regular program of crystal energetic healing.

Begin by wearing or carrying a programmed blue kyanite crystal. A rough, inexpensive piece is just as effective as something more elaborate when it comes to energy work. Follow with weekly crystal energy healing sessions, using the layout shown here. Program the crystals by asking:

> "I call upon the Light (or earth energies), please envelop these crystals with the highest vibration of peace, Light, strength, and positivity for the energy healing of (full name). I thank the Light.'

Fig. 59. The energy of obsessive compulsive disorder (OCD)

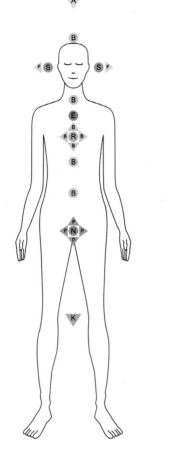

A =	ignitor crystal	12 inches (30 cm) above the crown chakra
B =	rose quartz	1 inch (2.5 cm) above crown chakra
S =	2 pyrite	3–6 inches (8–15 cm) beyond the ears
F =	2 clear quartz	single-terminated (directed outward) beyond the pyrite
B =	rose quartz	throat chakra
E =	blue kyanite	thymus (halfway between the throat and heart chakras)
R =	fluorite	heart chakra
B =	4 rose quartz	single-terminated (directed outward) around the fluorite on the heart chakra
B =	rose quartz	solar plexus chakra
B =	rose quartz	sacral chakra
N =	ruby	base chakra
P =	4 amethyst	single-terminated (directed outward) around the ruby on the base chakra
K =	exit crystal	between the knees

Crystal energy healing time: 10 minutes
Aftercare: rest, drink water, and (if time allows) bathe or shower
Repeat session: weekly.

The energy of bulimia

In cases where there is a pattern of food denial or food intolerance, soul recall therapy is an excellent way of accessing the energetic source of the difficulty and achieving some understanding of it. Clues will be revealed as to how to heal the energy of a person suffering with bulimia. From an energetic perspective, this condition is a rejection of self, life, and flow, with the energy of the sufferer being divided: a love of life on the one hand and a hatred of it on the other. This manifests in a pattern of behavior that takes the form of binge/expel/binge/expel, and this chaotic energy requires urgent rebalancing. Wearing or carrying a programmed blue kyanite crystal aligns and strengthens the physical energy body. A configuration of chakra balancing crystals (with some additions) can be used as shown. Program the crystals by asking:

> *"I call upon the Light (or earth energies), please envelop these crystals with the highest energetic vibration of peace, balance, harmony, and positivity for the energy healing of (full name). I thank the Light."*

Fig. 60. The energy of bulimia

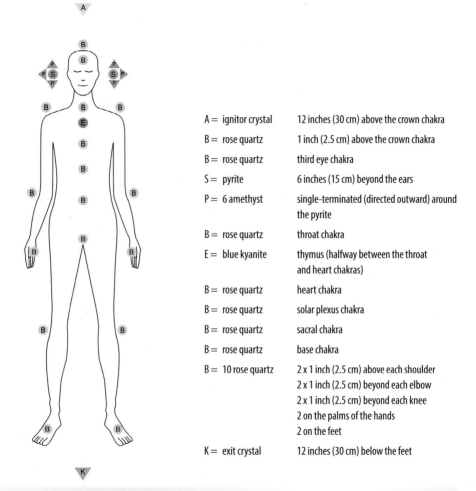

A =	ignitor crystal	12 inches (30 cm) above the crown chakra
B =	rose quartz	1 inch (2.5 cm) above the crown chakra
B =	rose quartz	third eye chakra
S =	pyrite	6 inches (15 cm) beyond the ears
P =	6 amethyst	single-terminated (directed outward) around the pyrite
B =	rose quartz	throat chakra
E =	blue kyanite	thymus (halfway between the throat and heart chakras)
B =	rose quartz	heart chakra
B =	rose quartz	solar plexus chakra
B =	rose quartz	sacral chakra
B =	rose quartz	base chakra
B =	10 rose quartz	2 x 1 inch (2.5 cm) above each shoulder
		2 x 1 inch (2.5 cm) beyond each elbow
		2 x 1 inch (2.5 cm) beyond each knee
		2 on the palms of the hands
		2 on the feet
K =	exit crystal	12 inches (30 cm) below the feet

Crystal energy healing time: 10 minutes
Aftercare: rest, drink water, and (if time allows) bathe or shower
Repeat session: weekly
Notes: secure the crystals onto areas such as the feet and the palms of the hands with microporous tape.

The energy of anorexia

From an energy perspective, anorexia is a denial of life, a cutting off from life, an inability to cope, and an inability to express, all of which bring about a spiraling negative energy. Once again, past life roots can be explored via soul recall therapy. Programmed kyanite worn or carried will strengthen and align the energy field. A programmed rose quartz will promote a higher connection to self-worth. The damaged energy field means that an anorexic lacks visual clarity. What they see is more or greater than what is in front of them. They see with the energy of loathing and then deny themselves. Crystal energy work can help the sufferer to move toward an energy of greater clarity. Regular chakra balancing crystals with some additions, as shown, can strengthen the energy field and help bring energetic healing to the chakra system. Great care must be taken, since the energy of the sufferer will be particularly weak and fragile. Crystals can be programmed by asking:

"I call upon the Light (or earth energies), please envelop these crystals with the highest energetic vibration of peace, balance, harmony, and positivity for the energy healing of (full name). I thank the Light."

Fig. 61. The energy of anorexia

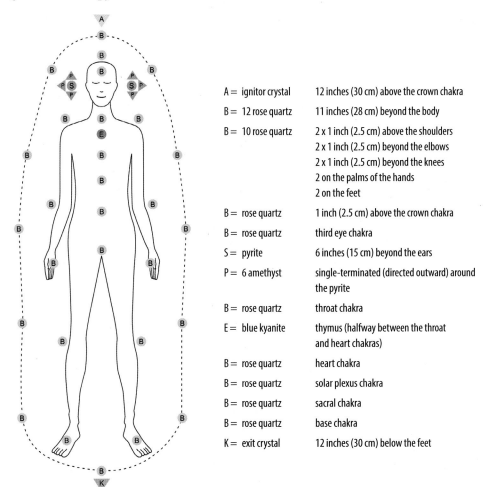

A =	ignitor crystal	12 inches (30 cm) above the crown chakra
B =	12 rose quartz	11 inches (28 cm) beyond the body
B =	10 rose quartz	2 x 1 inch (2.5 cm) above the shoulders
		2 x 1 inch (2.5 cm) beyond the elbows
		2 x 1 inch (2.5 cm) beyond the knees
		2 on the palms of the hands
		2 on the feet
B =	rose quartz	1 inch (2.5 cm) above the crown chakra
B =	rose quartz	third eye chakra
S =	pyrite	6 inches (15 cm) beyond the ears
P =	6 amethyst	single-terminated (directed outward) around the pyrite
B =	rose quartz	throat chakra
E =	blue kyanite	thymus (halfway between the throat and heart chakras)
B =	rose quartz	heart chakra
B =	rose quartz	solar plexus chakra
B =	rose quartz	sacral chakra
B =	rose quartz	base chakra
K =	exit crystal	12 inches (30 cm) below the feet

Crystal energy healing time: 10 minutes
Aftercare: rest, drink water, and (if time allows) bathe or shower
Repeat session: weekly until there is an alignment in strength
Notes: secure the crystals onto areas such as the feet and the palms of the hands with microporous tape.

The energy of cancer

Some people say that because energy is invisible it does not exist. It is the experience of many, including energy workers, that whether energy is seen, sensed, or felt, they know that it exists in and around the body. Just because we cannot see it, it does not mean that energy is not present.

As our main source of life, we cannot see the air that allows us to breathe. Energy is the same; it is within us and around us. If we now accept that, like air, energy surrounds us, it is also important to acknowledge that it plays a key role in everything we do, and in our health, whether good or poor. A blockage in our energy portals (chakras) or around us may come from energy blocks such as worry or physical injuries. This then extends in a number of ways. If, for example, we have constant dis-ease of our energy (worry, trauma, and so on), it can form a negative pool of energy in our individual energy field. This may occur around the chakras or in the general field of our energy. Like a pool of water that does not move or flow, this energy will eventually become stagnant. It will then progress and become denser in its form, settling closer into the physical energy. For instance, if you have experienced some kind of mental trauma that stagnates within your being, that energy will not be able to flow because you cannot move beyond it, and so in turn it evolves into stagnant energy that moves into the physical and emotional energy bands. Many people agree that mental ill health can cause a number of physical ailments, and it is acknowledged that worry and stress can bring on a heart attack. Something as seemingly simple as a rash can appear after a traumatic event, but all of these outcomes are serious enough to cause negative energy to build up in your energy field, and if they are not taken care of at an early stage, this energy can lay dormant and eventually become part of your physical being. It is as important to keep your energy in good health as it is your physical well-being. Whatever the cause of an ailment, it has an energy attached to it, and so it follows that with all cancers there will be an energy that can be worked on to help stimulate flow in the energy field once more. This can be seen as a preventative way to help heal the ailment in the energy field.

Once the cancer has taken hold and is in the physical body, it must be dealt with in a physical way, but if the body is healed from an energy perspective alongside treatment from a physician, then working on the energy field in conjunction with medical treatment will help recovery. It is important that energy is kept free-flowing since, as with all ailments, the dis-ease will be connected to a block in the energy field. Ensuring that energy flows will encourage good health, whether physical, emotional, mental, and, of course, spiritual. It is the aim of this book to help good energy practice achieve good energy health.

The energy of cancer (single site)*

Wearing rose quartz over the heart chakra brings the energy of peace and calm, together with the beginnings of greater positive energetic flow to the energy field. Introduce crystal chakra balancing for the cleansing and replenishing of positive energy to the energy field. Then follow the crystal layout for cancer (single site), which helps disperse the emotional holding of negative energy. Program the crystals by asking:

> *"I call upon the Light (or the earth energies), please envelop these crystals with the highest vibration of peace, Light, strength, and positivity for the energy healing of (full name). I thank the Light."*

* **For all health challenges please seek advice from a physical doctor to go hand in hand with the energy therapy you undertake.**

Fig. 62. The energy of cancer (single site)

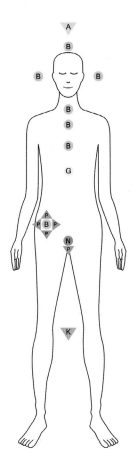

A =	ignitor crystal	4 inches (10 cm) above the crown chakra
B =	rose quartz	4 inches (10 cm) above the crown chakra
B =	2 rose quartz	4 inches (10 cm) beyond the ears
B =	rose quartz	throat chakra
B =	rose quartz	thymus (halfway between the throat and heart chakras)
B =	rose quartz	heart chakra
G =	rhodochrosite	solar plexus chakra
B =	rose quartz	centered to the site of the "dis-ease"
P =	4 amethyst	single-terminated (directed outward) around the rose quartz
N =	ruby	base chakra
P =	1 amethyst	single-terminated (directed downward) beneath the ruby
K =	exit crystal	between the knees

Crystal energy healing time: 10 minutes
Aftercare: rest, drink water, and (if time allows) bathe or shower
Repeat session: weekly for a month, then twice a month as required
Notes: when laying out base chakra crystals on the body, it is helpful for purposes of placement, removal, and the preservation of dignity, to first place a thick towel on the relevant part of the body.

The energy of cancer (multiple sites)*

From an energy perspective, the manifestation of cancer in different sites in the body is never random. Each site will have a key indicative factor for the puzzle that is the root cause energy. If you work with someone who is willing to pursue the metaphysical understanding of the disease, the crystal layouts will help you to understand how you can help their whole energy field. The layout shown here is for a person suffering with leukemia, where there is a great conflict of energy throughout the whole body. The use of rose quartz offers the ultimate energy of peace to assuage the energy of the inner turmoil. Program the crystals by asking:

> "I call upon the Light (or earth energies), please envelop these crystals with the highest vibration of peace, Light, strength, and positivity for the energy healing of (full name). I thank the Light."

For this particular energy healing, the volume of healing energy needs to be turned down in order not to encourage cell development, whether negative or positive. Without the ignitor and exit crystals, this energy healing is both a gentler process and a more positive experience for the recipient.

* For all health challenges please seek advice from a physical doctor to go hand in hand with the energy therapy you undertake.

Fig. 63. The energy of cancer (multiple sites)

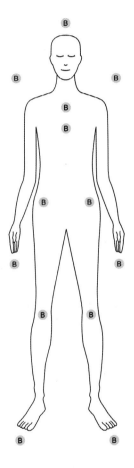

B =	rose quartz	4 inches (10 cm) above the crown chakra
B =	2 rose quartz	4 inches (10 cm) above the shoulders
B =	rose quartz	thymus (halfway between the throat and heart chakras)
B =	rose quartz	heart chakra
B =	rose quartz	hip bones
B =	2 rose quartz	4 inches (10 cm) beyond the middle fingers of the hands
B =	rose quartz	knees
B =	rose quartz	4 inches (10 cm) below the feet

Crystal energy healing time: 10 minutes
Aftercare: rest, drink water, and (if time allows) bathe or shower
Repeat session: weekly for a month, then twice a month as required
Notes: for gentle energy healing where there is conflict throughout the body, rose quartz offers the ultimate energy of peace. Take your time and use flowing movements to slowly position and remove the crystals in this kind of energy healing session. No ignitor and exit crystals are required as outlined.

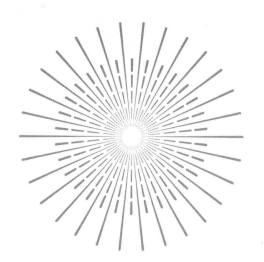

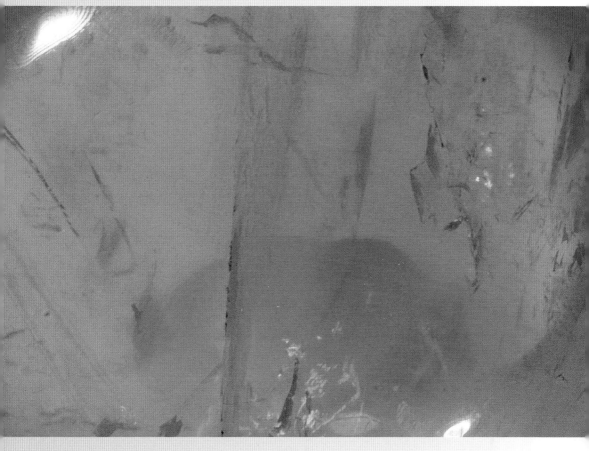

Chapter 11

Crystal Layouts
for Life
Enhancement

The energy of peace

True peace is rarely experienced in life. True peace has a vibrational quality that can reset our energetic clock, recalibrate us to our Light vibration, and take us back to our "Light factory settings," so to speak. True peace is like a stasis, a literal pause of energy, a state of pure equilibrium from which we can—almost—experience a rebirth. Shamans, wise peoples in our planet's history, ancient cultures, eastern cultures (where energy is not denied in the way that it is in the west) have through the ages valued the prize of true vibrational peace very highly—the ultimate of ultimates. They have experienced and truly understood its worth. Never has there been a time on our planet when we have needed to *be* of peace more than we do right now.

The ultimate bringer of peace, the crystal that imbues the greatest vibration of peace, is rose quartz. It is ubiquitous by Light design. It is relatively inexpensive and we are blessed that it is available to the many and not the few.

Wear or carry rose quartz programmed by asking:

"I call upon the Light (or earth energies), please charge this/these crystal/s with the highest positive energy to imbue (full name) with the energetic vibration of the Light of peace. I thank the Light."

This layout can be set out on a table or alternatively on the floor, allowing you enough room to sit or lie within the configuration. With floor configurations I find that if I roll out a yoga mat and place the crystals around it and then simply step into the layout and sit or lie down, I am already in the center, exactly where I need to be, with the mat as my body placement guide. Crystals can be programmed by asking:

"I call upon the Light, (or earth energies), please charge this/these crystal/s with highest positive energy to imbue (full name) with the energetic vibration of the Light of peace. I thank the Light."

Fig. 64. The energy of peace

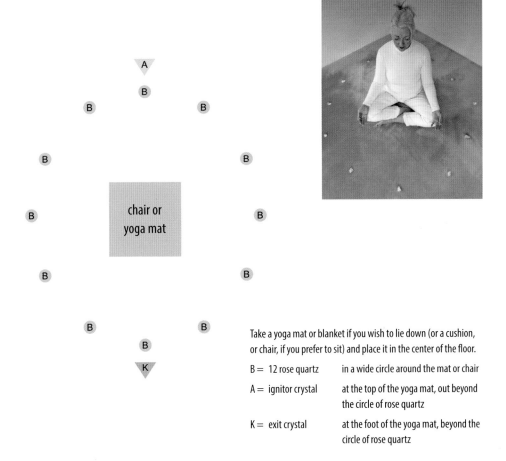

Take a yoga mat or blanket if you wish to lie down (or a cushion, or chair, if you prefer to sit) and place it in the center of the floor.

B =	12 rose quartz	in a wide circle around the mat or chair
A =	ignitor crystal	at the top of the yoga mat, out beyond the circle of rose quartz
K =	exit crystal	at the foot of the yoga mat, beyond the circle of rose quartz

Crystal energy healing time: 10 minutes
Aftercare: rest, drink water, and (if time allows) bathe or shower
Repeat session: weekly
Notes: this energy of peace layout/grid can also be arranged in a tighter tabletop formation (to sit before) for the duration of the session.

The energy of vitality

Vitality is an empowerment of physical energy, a life force energy that pervades the whole of the energy field. The energy of vitality is generous and effusive in nature, with a quality of empowerment, a can-do energy that "gives out," since the fountain from which this energy comes never stops if you continue to *pass on* the energy of your vitality, to give, with joy and positivity. To encourage vitality to enter your life in its truest energetic essence, program blue kyanite to wear or carry by asking:

> *"I call upon the Light (or earth energies), please charge this crystal with the highest positive energy to imbue (full name) with the energetic vibration of Light vitality. I thank the Light."*

Note: Blue kyanite is a master crystal that is unique in one particular respect: it does not require energy cleansing. Its self-cleansing property means that it perpetually cleanses and realigns its own being. Having said that, I do like to cleanse all my crystals and recommend that you do the same.

Fig. 65. The energy of vitality

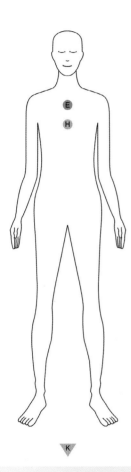

A = ignitor crystal   12 inches (30 cm) above the crown chakra

E = blue kyanite   thymus (halfway between the throat and heart chakras)

H = carnelian   heart chakra

K = exit crystal   12 inches (30 cm) below the feet

Crystal energy healing time: 10 minutes
Aftercare: rest, drink water, and (if time allows) bathe or shower
Repeat session: weekly as required
Notes: wear/carry a programmed kyanite between sessions.

The energy of abundance

Abundance in our dense physical realm usually suggests a significant amount of money. Money is merely energy, after all. However, it is important to remember that true energetic abundance takes many forms: love, support, opportunity, friendship, food on the table, a roof over your head, many gifts that we all too often take for granted. And these are in perfect harmonious flow, harmonious because the connections arrive in the right form at the right time for you in your life plan so that you can achieve what you elected to achieve when you were in the Light, prior to your incarnation on Earth. Being a coconspirator with the energy of abundance oils the wheels, so to speak, because you are working *with* the energy, and not *against* it; you are engaged with the purpose for being and not idling at the side of the road, looking the wrong way. To encourage the positive vibration of true abundance into your life, wear or carry a fluorite programmed by asking:

"I call upon the Light (or earth energies), please charge this/these crystal/s with the highest positive energy to facilitate the energy vibration of Light abundance into the life of (full name). I thank the Light."

Fig. 66. The energy of abundance (table layout)

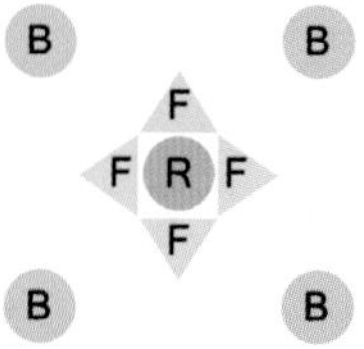

R = fluorite — center of layout

F = 4 clear quartz — single-terminated (directed outward) around the fluorite

B = 4 rose quartz — in a square formation around the clear quartz (as shown)

Fig. 67. The energy of abundance (body layout)

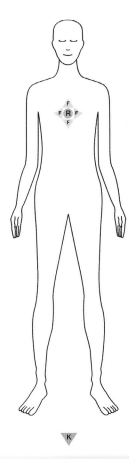

A = ignitor crystal   12 inches (30 cm) above the crown chakra

R = fluorite   heart chakra

F = 4 clear quartz   single-terminated (directed outward) around the fluorite

K = exit crystal   12 inches (30 cm) below the feet

Crystal energy healing time: 10 minutes
Aftercare: rest, drink water, and (if time allows) bathe or shower
Repeat session: weekly as required
Notes: the energy of abundance layout/grid can be placed on the body as shown, or it can be configured as a tabletop layout (to sit before).

A personal gateway to the soul layout

This is a tabletop configuration of crystals that opens (and closes) an energy portal or gateway. This is the vehicle that allows you to connect with greater clarity to your higher self, masters, guides, and angels in the Light, among others, in order to reattune, realign, and

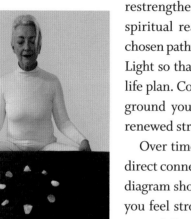

restrengthen (via a Light connection directly from the spiritual realm of your higher consciousness) on your chosen pathway. Remember, you chose this pathway in the Light so that you could achieve it on Earth through your life plan. Connecting to the Light in this way helps you to ground your Light to the Earth through your body in renewed strength toward this energy of achievement.

Over time, using the crystals allows you to establish a direct connection to your intuition and open up to it. The diagram shows a basic gateway layout/grid, but if in time you feel strongly about introducing another crystal that powerfully resonates with you, include the new crystal (as a pair) by replacing the turquoise, for example, as shown.

Follow your heart on your choice of crystal. The rose quartz and turquoise are the crystals to change, if any, in the configuration, as the clear quartz crystal and the snow quartz form an alchemical energetic framework to this particular layout. If you choose an alternative, do stick with it because you are creating an energetic key. It functions like any other key and the door is *your* gateway to *your* higher self. It is important that you both respect and protect this. Practice it and you will strengthen your own personal key; the door to your higher self will open, becoming a powerful place for you to meditate.

Ten minutes a week is a good way to begin. Remember that a lot can happen in ten minutes when you are connecting to your higher self (linear time only exists on Earth and beyond Earth you are on the

Fig. 68. The energy of wisdom

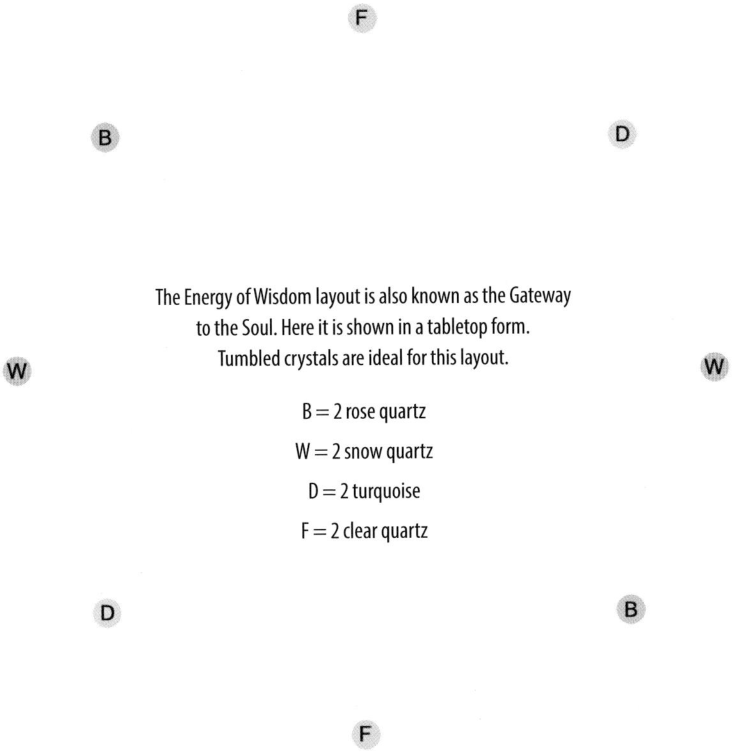

F

B   D

W   W

The Energy of Wisdom layout is also known as the Gateway
to the Soul. Here it is shown in a tabletop form.
Tumbled crystals are ideal for this layout.

B = 2 rose quartz

W = 2 snow quartz

D = 2 turquoise

F = 2 clear quartz

D   B

F

Crystal energy healing time: 10 minutes
Aftercare: rest, drink water, and (if time allows) bathe or shower
Repeat session: weekly as required
Notes: with practice, the Energy of Wisdom layout/grid is a useful tool for connecting to
your higher self and your accumulated wisdom. It is a powerful session, so take time to align
yourself afterward. Remember that having a drink of water and a little light food helps to
ground the body following deep crystal energy healing and/or meditation.

cosmic clock). How often you wish to continue is up to you. Many people use this method as a platform to develop and strengthen a continuing connection to the Light. Cleanse the crystals before you start, lay them out as shown, open the energy ("I call upon the Light [or earth energies], please open the energy to my personal crystal configuration at this time. I thank the Light."), meditate, and then close the energy ("I call upon the Light [or earth energies], please close the energy of my personal crystal configuration at this time. I thank the Light."). Cleanse the crystals and put them away. I keep mine in a velvet bag, stored in a drawer. Crystals can be programmed before use by asking:

> "I call upon the Light, (or the earth energies) please charge these crystals with the highest positivity that they may connect me to my higher self. I thank the Light."

A–Z of key crystals
to use in crystal circuits

Abalone

Healing focus: a bone and skeletal strengthener.

Crystal layout use: place on the center of
fractures or breaks to promote energy healing.

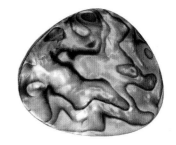

Amber

Healing focus: opens the heart energy and settles
the emotions. Place over the heart chakra.

Crystal layout use: incorporate into a crystal
circuit for anxiety and fearfulness.

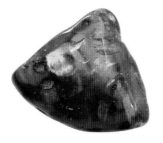

Amethyst

Healing focus: the stone of transmutation and
spiritual connection. A powerful energy protector.

Crystal layout use: place on the solar plexus
chakra to release emotional holding and
strengthen the energy field.

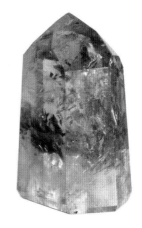

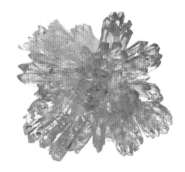

Amethyst chrysanthemum

Healing focus: opens and strengthens the crown chakra. Enhances spiritual connection to the Light.

Crystal layout use: place 12 inches (30 cm) above the crown chakra.

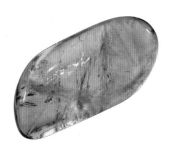

Ametrine

Healing focus: a gentle purifier of the sinuses, which are connected with blocked energy related to the family.

Crystal layout use: place over energy blocks on the head or face to achieve release.

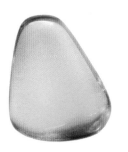

"Andara crystal" (blue obsidian, artificial)

Healing focus: the communication crystal. Promotes the energy of positive clarity in dealings with other people.

Crystal layout use: place on the throat chakra to promote clarity of communication and connection with those around you.

"Apache Tear" (obsidian)

Healing focus: the grief crystal. Resolves the energy of pain and loss.

Crystal layout use: gently place one crystal beneath each eye to help alleviate grief.

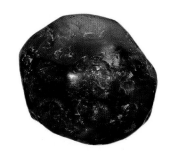

"Aqua aura quartz" (treated clear quartz)

Healing focus: encourages higher connection to the Light and promotes unconditional love in action.

Crystal layout use: place on the heart chakra to open and strenghten this key chakra.

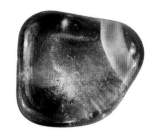

Aquamarine

Healing focus: draws higher etheric Light and promotes intuitive creativity (throat chakra).

Crystal layout use: apply to the throat chakra to cleanse or release energy blocks.

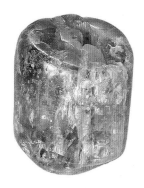

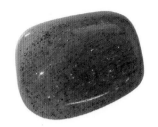

Aventurine quartz

Healing focus: moves us toward the Light strength of individuality and self-determination in order to forge our own path in life.

Crystal layout use: place on the sacral chakra to inspire greater confidence in the timid.

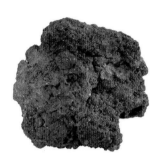

Azurite

Healing focus: promotes clarity of communication in families, social or professional groups, and business.

Crystal layout use: place on the solar plexus and throat chakras to release buried trauma.

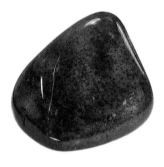

"Bloodstone" (heliotrope)

Healing focus: a bringer of earth energy. A grounding stone for the sacral chakra.

Crystal layout use: place on the sacral chakra to help those who are ungrounded.

Boji stone

Healing focus: a balancer of the heart and solar plexus chakras.

Crystal layout use: place on the heart and solar plexus to bring equilibrium to any bullying or overpowering energy and to promote greater compassion.

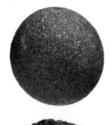
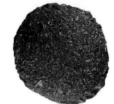

Calcite (pink)

Healing focus: helps to overcome an energetic challenge with empowerment and enhances calm.

Crystal layout use: applied within crystal circuitry to areas of great pain.

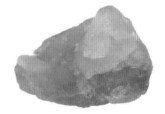

Calcite (mangano calcite)

Healing focus: a higher/angelic connector to overcome extremes of pain.

Crystal layout use: helps with intense pain, whether physical, emotional, mental, or spiritual.

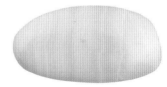

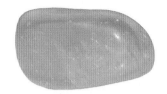

Calcite (yellow)

Healing focus: draws the energy of the sun (joy).

Crystal layout use: place on the third eye chakra for low mood or pessimism.

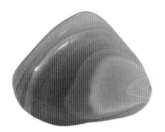

Carnelian

Healing focus: a purification stone for the sacral chakra.

Crystal layout use: place on the sacral chakra for those who lack vibrancy and joy.

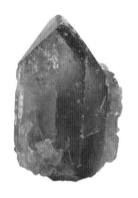

Celestite

Healing focus: facilitates connection to all streams of angelic consciousness.

Crystal layout use: place on the thymus chakra of a chronically ill person to promote peace.

Chalcedony

Healing focus: delivers spiritual connection.
Crystal layout use: place 2 inches (5 cm) above
the crown chakra for difficult life path choices.

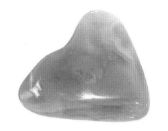

Chalcopyrite (gold in color)

Healing focus: absorbs stubborn, stagnant,
negative patterns from the energy field.
Crystal layout use: in crystal circuitry place
9 inches (23 cm) from the ears to help overcome
negative habits.

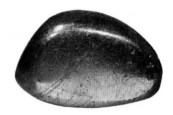

Chiastolite "the cross-stone"

Healing focus: promotes awareness to the
ascension path.
Crystal layout use: place on the sacral chakra
in crystal circuitry for obsessions with the minor
things in life.

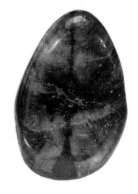

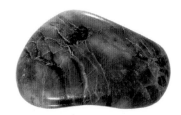

Chrysocolla

Healing focus: a connector to divine light.
A spiritual strengthener.

Crystal layout use: place an inch away from the
hands of those suffering with a chronic illness.

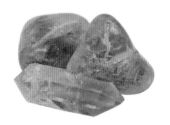

Citrine

Healing focus: an energetic cleanser and purifier.
A bringer of joy and vitality.

Crystal layout use: place on the solar plexus
chakra to ignite more enthusiasm for life.

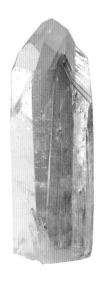

Clear quartz

Healing focus: radiates pure Light energy and
holds the full spectrum of vibrational rays.

Crystal layout use: place an inch above the crown
chakra for energetic detoxification.

Clear quartz (the ignitor crystal)

Healing focus: the charge crystal in circuitry. A bringer of pure Light energy to cleanse and positivize.

Crystal layout use: position the body of the person being treated (or your own) between the ignitor and exit crystals for a cleansing energy recharge.

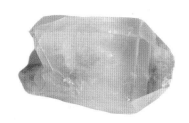

Clear quartz (orb)

Healing focus: promotes connection to cosmic energy. A very powerful meditation tool.

Crystal layout use: sit with the orb, a rose quartz crystal in each hand, to magnify the energy of peace.

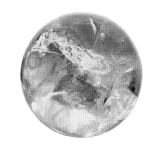

Clear quartz (single-terminated point)

Healing focus: radiates pure Light energy with a single directional focus.

Crystal layout use: amplifies and directs the energy of a different crystal.

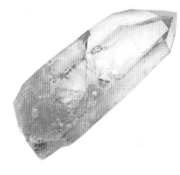

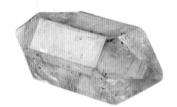

Clear quartz (double-terminated point)

Healing focus: radiates pure Light energy with a double directional focus.

Crystal layout use: turns up the volume of the pull between crystals in a multi-crystal layout.

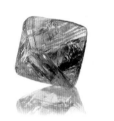

Diamond

Healing focus: the manifestation of the Light, and of the strength, perfection, and vibration of all the healing rays.

Crystal layout use: jewelry can be programmed and charged to positivize the energy field.

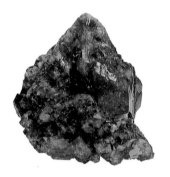

Dioptase

Healing focus: brings fulfilment.

Crystal layout use: place on the heart chakra for greater self-empowerment.

Emerald

Healing focus: clears the vision and heals the heart. A cellular regenerator. Balances the four lower bodies.

Crystal layout use: place on the heart chakra for loss of energy.

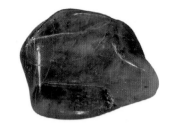

Fluorite

Healing focus: overcomes emotional pain, delivers strength for a difficult life path, and releases karma.

Crystal layout use: place on any site on the body where flow is blocked.

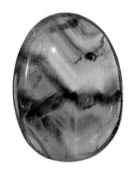

Garnet

Healing focus: purifies the base chakra.

Crystal layout use: place on the base chakra for anger issues.

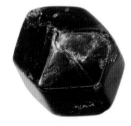

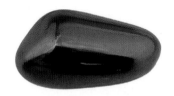

Hematite

Healing focus: purifies life force (blood) and grounds energy to the earth.

Crystal layout use: place on the base chakra to combat toxins.

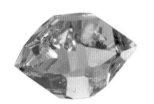

"Herkimer diamond" (clear quartz)

Healing focus: promotes strength and prosperity.

Crystal layout use: place on both palm chakras to support the energy of abundant flow.

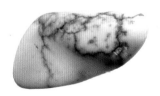

Howlite

Healing focus: supports mental energy and enhances attentiveness, retention, and the flow of knowledge.

Crystal layout use: place on the third eye chakra for woolly thinking.

Iceland spar

Healing focus: a gentle, continuous Light strengthener.

Crystal layout use: place on the solar plexus for those drained of energy.

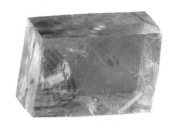

Jade (jadeite)

Healing focus: Promotes abundance and generosity (to use wisely and freely).

Crystal layout use: place on the heart chakra to encourage generosity of spirit.

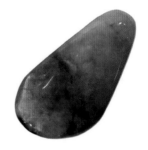

Jasper (red)

Healing focus: heals the spleen and strengthens the immune system.

Crystal layout use: place on the sacral chakra after illness or for diminished energy.

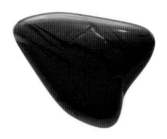

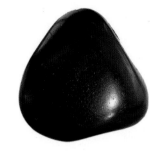

Jet

Healing focus: brings infinite energy and helps us to flow through the universe while strengthening our place within it.

Crystal layout use: place 12 inches (30 cm) above the crown chakra for life and career changes.

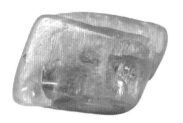

Kunzite

Healing focus: the connector of the heart to the Light. A relationship crystal. Promotes harmony.

Crystal layout use: place on the solar plexus to heal relationship issues.

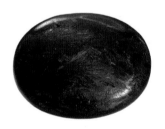

Kyanite (black)

Healing focus: connects and aligns to infinite possibilities for the soul.

Crystal layout use: place 12 inches (30 cm) above the crown chakra to combat a fear of the future.

Kyanite (blue)

Healing focus: a supreme energy aligner, cleanser, and balancer.

Crystal layout use: place on the thymus chakra to promote the alignment of energy.

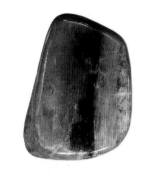

Kyanite (green)

Healing focus: helps to align the energy of physical matter. Realigns and rebalances.

Crystal layout use: place on the heart chakra for a physical energetic boost.

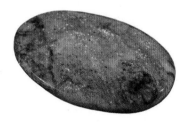

Labradorite

Healing focus: heals the thymus chakra and boosts the immune system.

Crystal layout use: place on the thymus chakra to strengthen the energy of the immune system.

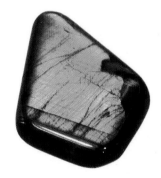

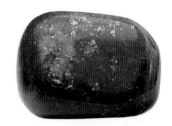

Lapis lazuli

Healing focus: promotes clear-sightedness (third eye chakra). Opens a Light channel to the divine self.

Crystal layout use: strengthens the connection to the Light by placing on the third eye chakra.

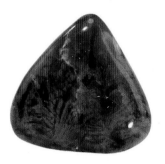

Luvulite (sugilite)

Healing focus: heals a suffering, troubled heart.

Crystal layout use: place on the heart chakra to bring the energy of peace and alignment to the heart and the strength to move forward.

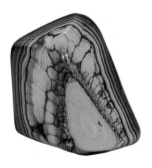

Malachite

Healing focus: soothes stress and emotional or mental turmoil. Heals the heart and calms the mind.

Crystal layout use: place on the heart chakra for anxiety.

Moldavite

Healing focus: brings connection to the universe.

Crystal layout use: hold in the right palm to raise consciousness and see the bigger picture.

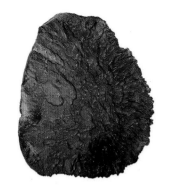

Moonstone

Healing focus: settles emotional hurt and helps with moving forward.

Crystal layout use: place on the solar plexus chakra to help heal the energy of an emotional wound.

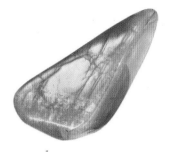

Obsidian "snowflake obsidian"

Healing focus: releases negativity. Promotes connection to the Light.

Crystal layout use: hold one crystal in each palm and position the body of the person being treated (or your own) between the ignitor and exit crystals, arranged in a circuit.

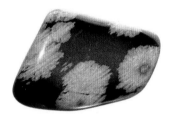

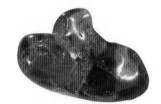

Opal "fire opal"

Healing focus: attracts the Light energy of positivity and joy.

Crystal layout use: place on the third eye chakra for depression.

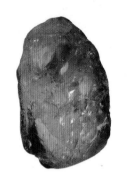

Peridot

Healing focus: an energizer stone to promote balance and harmony.

Crystal layout use: place on the center of the area of discomfort to support a sluggish digestive system.

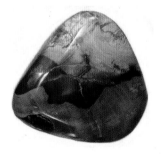

Petrified wood

Healing focus: a grounding energy to the earth and a connector to earth energy.

Crystal layout use: place on the sacral chakra to promote and develop intuitive ability to the mineral, plant, or animal kingdom.

Pyrite

Healing focus: absorbs negative electromagnetic energy and releases negative thinking patterns.

Crystal layout use: place 8 inches (20 cm) above the crown chakra.

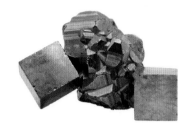

Rhodochrosite

Healing focus: calms emotional pain and promotes peace and harmony.

Crystal layout use: place on the solar plexus for deep-seated emotional wounds.

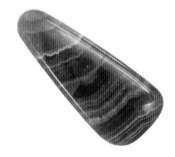

Rose quartz

Healing focus: bringer of peace and energy healing. Resonates to skin energy healing.

Crystal layout use: place on the site of discomfort for chronic pain.

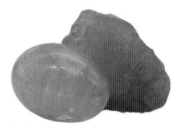

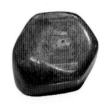

Ruby

Healing focus: a bringer of unconditional love (the ruby ray). Purifies the base (root) chakra.

Crystal layout use: use to release a blocked base chakra.

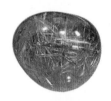

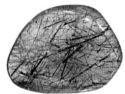

Rutilated quartz

Healing focus: the mending stone for skeletal breaks and bone weakness disorders.

Crystal layout use: place on the sacral chakra for strength to face a challenging life.

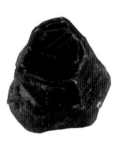

Sapphire

Healing focus: purifies throat energy.

Crystal layout use: use on the throat chakra for suppressed or anger energy.

Selenite

Healing focus: heals skin and digestive flow.
A cellular regenerator.

Crystal layout use: use on skin flares or digestive
blocks.

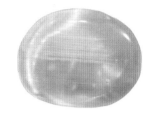

Smoky quartz

Healing focus: an absorber of negative energy.

Crystal layout use: hold one crystal in each palm
between the ignitor and exit crystals, in circuit, to
release control issues.

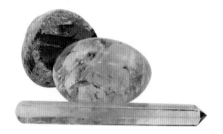

Smoky quartz (the exit crystal)

Healing focus: the absorber crystal in circuitry.
Facilitates transmutation of negative energy.

Crystal layout use: program to cleanse the four
lower bodies and sit before the exit crystal for
10 minutes.

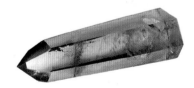

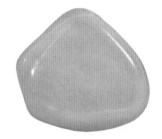

Snow quartz

Healing focus: an angelic connector. Heals and protects the sacral chakra.

Crystal layout use: hold one crystal in each palm to nurture strength and intuition.

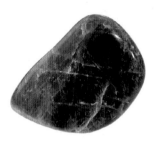

Sodalite

Healing focus: heals the throat chakra (following misuse of the throat chakra). A truth in life stone.

Crystal layout use: use on the throat chakra for habitual smoking issues.

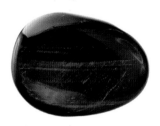

Tiger's eye (blue)

Healing focus: heals negativity in blocks to speaking.

Crystal layout use: place on the throat chakra to promote confidence and flow.

Tiger's eye (gold)

Healing focus: heals the negativity in a lack of clarity and clear-sightedness. Clears vision that has been clouded by energy.

Crystal layout use: place on the third eye chakra to connect to the energy of higher clarity, positivity, and wisdom.

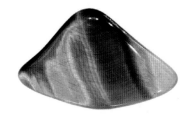

Topaz (blue)

Healing focus: enhances clarity of sight, speech, and communication for the beauty of the spiritual self.

Crystal layout use: use on the third eye, throat, and heart chakras for greater self-belief.

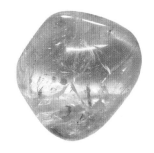

Topaz (gold)

Healing focus: promotes clarity of mind and greater mental focus. Attunes to higher wisdom.

Crystal layout use: place on the third eye chakra to clear fogginess.

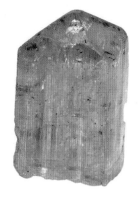

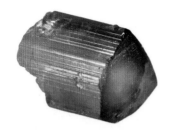

Tourmaline (green)

Healing focus: promotes balance, harmony, and flow to physical energy.

Crystal layout use: place on the heart chakra to help with depletion or obsessive thinking.

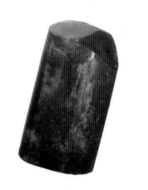

Tourmaline (pink)

Healing focus: supports balanced emotional energy.

Crystal layout use: place on the heart chakra for highly charged feelings and extremes of emotion.

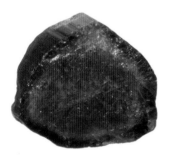

Tourmaline "watermelon tourmaline"

Healing focus: brings balance to the four lower bodies.

Crystal layout use: place on the heart chakra to overcome challenges or weakness.

Turquoise

Healing focus: promotes connection to higher consciousness and greater spiritual awareness.

Crystal layout use: place on the third eye and heart chakras for stages of grief.

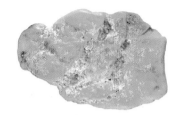

Unakite

Healing focus: the "team stone" that promotes common unity. Encourages harmony and balance.

Crystal layout use: hold a crystal in each palm between the ignitor and exit crystals, in circuit, to promote harmony.

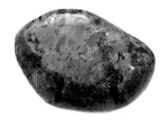

Glossary of terms

Active crystal A crystal in use.

Alchemy Transmutational change for the positive.

Alignment ("A-line-to-Light") Developing constant awareness, connection, and flow in action with and in Light.

Assumption A belief spoken, born of the mind.

Aura The energy field that surrounds any living entity, which is also rooted within their physical vehicle (body).

Call To invoke the Light with focus.

Cellular imprint A place on the body carrying a particular focus of soul patterning, such as a past life war wound.

Cellular memory The pattern of the soul plan (past, present, and potential). Held within each cell of our bodies, it may be activated by date, place, or personal connection.

Chakra Sanskrit for "spinning wheel," a vortex of Light within and without the energy field.

Circuit A grid of crystals that make up an energy pattern for a particular healing purpose (see *Crystal circuits*).

Clairaudient "Clear-hearing" with intuition.

Clairsentient "Clear-feeling" with intuition.

Clairvoyant "Clear-seeing" with intuition.

Cleansing To release accumulated held negativity that has been absorbed by a crystal.

Closing (energy) To cease a healing session.

Crystal absorption The capacity and quantity of negative energy that a crystal can draw from a being or place.

Crystal cairn An environmental structure with a crystal on the top to promote positive energy focus.

Crystal circuits Patterns or grids of energy for a healing charge of focus, usually with an ignitor crystal and an exit crystal to empower the circuit.

Crystal therapist An experienced practitioner using crystals to enhance the lives of others in connection to the soul.

Directing energy "Pointing" energy with intent.

Dis-ease The energy of non-alignment that gathers over time, becoming an area of negative energy, first outside the body in the energy field, and then making its way into the body.

Divine matrix The "perfect" you, the pattern of you according to God's will. The focus toward which we should all strive.

Dormant crystal A crystal not in use.

Earth energy Your connection to earth, a grounding energy that allows you to release your karmic energy.

Egg A solid mass of crystal that is usually egg-shaped, with a special healing capacity.

Energy The life force within and without (inside and outside) any living entity.

Energy "attraction" The magnetism of the life force, whether crystals or human beings.

Gem bathing Using gem elixirs to drop into your bath so that you can enjoy the vibrational healing of the crystal.

Gem elixirs A remedy made from a Light charge that is emitted from a crystal.

Hands on To apply your hands as a conduit of Light for the divine.

Healing To cleanse, transmute, and eradicate negative energy and bring to flow energetic beauty, harmony, and positivity.

Healing energy To apply the positive flow of the Light to another person or yourself.

Holistic reflexology To practice reflexology in acknowledgment of the whole being, so that the body is being treated as well as the human energy field.

Human energy field The four lower bodies that make up the human energy system of greatest importance for our health.

Hypnosis A method of controlling another person's mental energy.

Ignited crystal A crystal in use with focus or charged for a particular healing purpose.

Igniting Light charging a crystal for a particular healing purpose.

Ignitor crystal The charge crystal in a crystal circuit; it empowers the circuit.

Intention A direction of your energy.

Intuition ("Inner – tuition") Your inner sense and knowing; it comes from your connection to your life plan/guides, by which you are prompted.

Intuitive response To work with the energy of intuition toward healing another person in connection with your divine knowledge and guides.

Journey of the soul The progressive learning experience of the soul from life to the Light, again and again, until they have ascended beyond and beyond and beyond.

Karma "As you sow, so shall you reap." The cosmic law of consequence, good or other.

Karmic energy The energy we carry to clear, apportioned to us each day.

Karmic responsibility A soul promise.

Life plan The predestined opportunities and tests chosen in the Light prior to life and lived out in the incarnation.

Light Divine energy.

Magnification (energy) To grow and expand energy.

Meditation To release negative energy, to connect to the divine, and to repositivize your whole being.

Meridian Part of the structure of the human Light body, whose function is to flow universal life force through the body and energy field.

Moon cleansing To place crystals in moonlight, allowing the moon's energy to wash them clean.

Orb A solid mass of crystal, usually round in appearance, with an empowered energy healing capacity.

Pain Resistant held energy.

Portals Energy gateways.

Positivizing (energy) To make good and of flow.

Primary energy Pure Light divine connection that moves down through the crown chakra.

Professional holistic healer/therapist A person who has dedicated themselves at a soul level to healing others.

Programming (crystals) Investing a focus of energy to a crystal that will, in turn, direct the energy in action. (Asking.)

Rays Divine Light streams of energy, blessed to Earth.

Sealing energy To protect your own Light and energy field or that of others.

Soul recall (or past life) therapist A therapist who facilitates connections to past life memory (or memories) in order to release current blocks to the present life plan via a meditative technique. (This is not hypnosis.)

Spirit Divine energy.

Spiritual connection To access the divine.

Sun cleansing To place a crystal in sunlight, allowing the sun's energy to wash it clean.

Tabular quartz crystal A crystal shaped like a lozenge or tablet, single- or double-terminated. When used as an ignitor or exit crystal in a crystal circuit, it is best to choose single-terminated tabular crystals.

Threefold energy system The combined energy system comprised of the primary energy coming down from the crown chakra, earth energy coming up from the feet and universal energy being drawn in by the chakra system.

Toolkit (crystals) A therapist's collection of crystals for the purpose of crystal healing.

Transmutation The true release of negative energy from someone or something and its release to earth, directed to flow now in positivity once more.

Universal energy Positive Light energy that is drawn in through the chakra system.

Index

Acknowledgments

There are many beings whom I would like to thank for their valued contribution toward bringing this book *Crystal Body Grids* into fruition. Please know that I thank you from my heart with deep appreciation and that I am truly grateful to each one of you.

In particular, I would like to thank my immediate family for their patience, love, support, and practical help: Cameron McAllister for transforming my diagrams into digital clarity and for providing additional photography; Stuart McAllister for his great positivity and infinite inspirational assistance; and also not forgetting Angus and Ruaraigh for offering their cheery encouragement together with endless cups of tea.

I thank each one of you from the depths of my heart.

Sharon L. McAllister

About the author

Sharon L. McAllister has been a holistic therapist for more than thirty years, specializing in reflexology, soul recall therapy, and crystal healing. Sharon lives and works in Scotland and has taught reflexology and crystal healing at both diploma and advanced level.

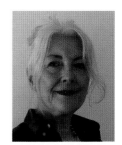

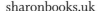

sharonbooks.uk

Picture credits

Crystal photographs by Karola Sieber, www.makrogalerie.de
Except the following:
Cameron McAllister: pp. 24, 177, back flap (ignitor crystal), p. 173 (pink calcite), p. 174 (celestite), p. 176 (citrine), p. 187 (rose quartz and pyrite), p. 189 (smoky quartz)
Shutterstock: p. 5–7: Nature's Charm, p. 11: ju_see, p. 24, 189 (exit crystal): Roy Palmer, p. 41: ju_see, p. 173 (mangano calcite): vvoe, pp. 177, back flap (single-terminated clear quartz): Mara Fribus, p. 183 (green kyanite) Hyperborean_treasures, p. 178, back flap (double-terminated clear quartz): William G Forbes

Crystal body grids photographs:
Cameron McAllister: p. 25, p. 44, p. 60, p. 78, p. 88, p. 100, p. 116, p. 142, p. 161, p. 166. Models: Sharon McAllister, Angus McAllister, Ruaraigh McAllister

Decorative designs throughout (light flashes): Liubou Yasiukovich/Shutter stock.com
Body diagrams throughout: Cameron McAllister, www.camer-on.uk
All drawings by Sharon McAllister

Also by Sharon McAllister

In **Awakening Your Crystals**, experienced holistic therapist and crystal-healing trainer Sharon L. McAllister shares not only what crystals can do for you but also how forging a connection to a crystal itself, treating it with respect and care, and programming it appropriately, will awaken its full powers and intensify your healing experience.

The practical information ranges from explaining the use of gemstones for yourself in everyday life to the responsible therapeutic treatment of others. Eight key crystals are portrayed, supported by vibrant photog- raphy, and form a toolkit that covers a dazzling array of applications. More than 60 additional crystals are described in an A–Z directory to give a complete overview of the diverse possibilities that gemstones offer us.

- Detailed guidance on programming crystals
- Quick reference to the healing properties of more than 60 crystals
- Includes relevant information for professional crystal therapists

Portraits of eight key crystals:
Rose Quartz, Amethyst, Pyrite, Celestite, Smoky Quartz, Citrine, Fluorite, Unakite

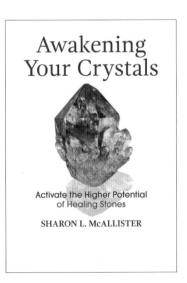

Awakening
Your Crystals

Activate the Higher Potential
of Healing Stones

SHARON L. McALLISTER

Sharon L. McAllister
Awakening Your Crystals
Activate the Higher Potential
of Healing Stones
Paperback, full-color throughout,
176 pages
ISBN 978-1-62055-972-7

Other books by Earthdancer

Healing Crystals is a comprehensive and up-to-date directory of 555 healing gemstones, presented in a practical and handy pocket guide format. In the revised edition of his bestseller, Michael Gienger, famous for his pioneering work in the field of crystal healing, describes the characteristics and healing powers of each crystal in a clear, concise, and precise style, accompanied by four-color photographs.

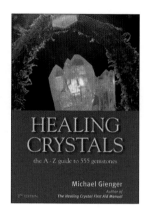

Michael Gienger
Healing Crystals
the A–Z guide to 555 gemstones, 2nd edition
Paperback, full-color throughout, 128 pages
ISBN 978-1-84409-647-3

Gem water can be a valuable aid to health, providing effective remedies and acting quickly on a physical level. Water is known to carry mineral information, so by placing crystals in water it becomes charged with the crystals' energy. Drinking gem water as a therapeutic treatment is similar and complementary to wearing crystals, although the effects are not necessarily the same. Gem Water should be prepared and used with care; this book explains everything you need to know to get started.

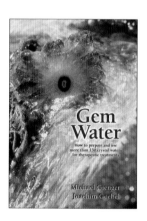

Michael Gienger, Joachim Goebel
Gem Water
How to prepare and use more than 130 crystal waters
for therapeutic treatments
Paperback, full-color throughout, 96 pages
ISBN 978-1-84409-131-7

Other books by Earthdancer

Tapping into children's seemingly inherent love of rocks and stones, this accessible introduction to gemology provides youngsters with a basic understanding of the properties that crystals possess, the power of color, and the metaphysical importance of positive thinking. Divided into seven sections, each chakra is explored and visualization exercises are included in order to experience the chakra's energy.

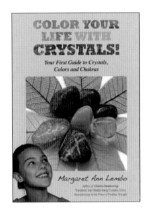

Margaret Ann Lembo
Color Your Life With Crystals
Your first guide to crystals, colors, and chakras
Paperback, full-color throughout, 112 pages
ISBN 978-1-84409-605-3

In this full-color guide, the authors explain how to calculate your personal numbers and work with the healing energies of gemstones to unfold the full potential your numbers reveal. The authors describe which crystals resonate most with each number's energy and offer affirmations, meditations, and crystal healing techniques to connect with gemstone energies.

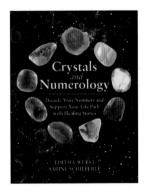

Editha Wuest, Sabine Schieferle
Crystals and Numerology
Decode Your Numbers and Support Your Life Path
with Healing Stones
Paperback, full-color throughout, 160 pages
ISBN 978-1-64411-273-1

Other books by Earthdancer

This useful little guidebook provides everything you need to know about cleansing crystals—including both the well-known and the less well-known methods. It clearly explains the best method for each purpose, whether for charging or discharging, cleansing on an external or energetic level, or eliminating foreign information.

Michael Gienger
Purifying Crystals
How to clear, charge, and purify your healing crystals
Paperback, full-color throughout, 64 pages
ISBN 978-1-84409-147-8

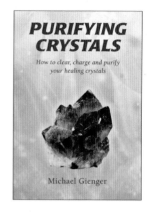

This pocket pharmacy of healing stones embraces many applications. Although describing only twelve stones, the breadth of its scope resembles a home pharmacy. From allergies to toothache, you will find the right stone for every application. This handy little book offers you the essence of our modern knowledge of healing stones.

Michael Gienger
Twelve Essential Healing Crystals
Your first aid manual for preventing and treating common ailments from allergies to toothache.
Paperback, full-color throughout, 64 pages
ISBN 978-1-84409-642-8

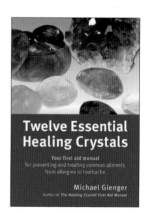

Other books by Earthdancer

This visually impressive book brings the reader up close to the beauty and diversity of the quartz crystal family. Its unique and concise presentation allows the reader to quickly and easily identify an array of quartz crystals and become familiar with their distinctive features and energetic properties.

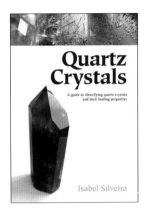

Isabel Silveira
Quartz Crystals
A guide to identifying quartz crystals and their healing properties
Paperback, full-color throughout, 80 pages
ISBN 978-1-84409-148-5

This is an easy-to-use A to Z guide for treating many common ailments and illnesses with the help of crystal therapy. It includes a comprehensive color appendix with photographs and short descriptions of each gemstone recommended.

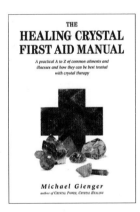

Michael Gienger
The Healing Crystal First Aid Manual
A practical A to Z of common ailments and illnesses and how they can be best treated with crystal therapy.
Paperback, with 16 color plates, 288 pages
ISBN 978-1-84409-084-6

For further information and to request a book catalog contact:
Inner Traditions, One Park Street, Rochester, Vermont 05767

Earthdancer Books is an Inner Traditions imprint.
Phone: +1-800-246-8648, customerservice@innertraditions.com
www.earthdancerbooks.com • www.innertraditions.com

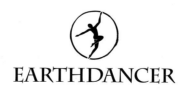

EARTHDANCER

AN INNER TRADITIONS IMPRINT